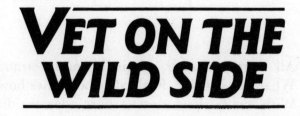

VET ON THE WILD SIDE

All things counter, original, spare, strange;
Whatever is fickle, freckled (who knows how?)
With swift, slow; sweet, sour; adazzle, dim;
He fathers-forth whose beauty is past change:
                              Praise him.
        Gerard Manley Hopkins, 'Pied Beauty'

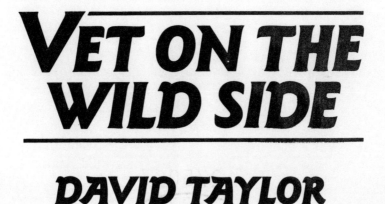

VET ON THE WILD SIDE

DAVID TAYLOR

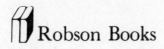
Robson Books

First published in Great Britain in 1990 by Robson Books Ltd,
Bolsover House, 5–6 Clipstone Street, London WIP 7EB

British Library Cataloguing in Publication Data

Taylor, David,
 Vet on the wild side.
 1. Great Britain. Veterinary medicine – Biographies
 I. Title
 636.0890922

ISBN 0 86051 660 1

Photoset by Rowland Phototypesetting Ltd,
Bury St Edmunds, Suffolk
Printed in Great Britain by
Butler and Tanner Ltd,
Frome, Somerset

To the memory of my father, Frank Taylor, of Diggle and Taylor's, Rochdale.

Contents

Introduction

As I write, it's almost exactly twenty years since I left general practice in Rochdale, Lancashire, to found the world's first independent, peripatetic veterinary service devoted exclusively to exotic animals. Since 1957 I had been working part-time with the once-great Belle Vue Zoo in Manchester, learning from people like Matt Kelly, the head keeper, many of the traditional ways of handling wild animals and coping with their illnesses. I'd also learned that, when I began, there was little in the way of dedicated zoological medicine, and meagre interest in aardvarks and axolotls, zebras and zorillas among veterinarians in general.

The world of an aspiring zoo vet was wide open, I realized, and awash with opportunities. New methods of safely controlling timid or dangerous beasts by means of flying syringes were just around the corner and about to revolutionize exotic animal management. The first safari parks and marinelands, housing new and exciting species, were being set up and they would demand new and exciting kinds of medicine.

So it was that I bade farewell to the old surgery on Milnrow Road, the two o'clock and seven o'clock consulting hours for dogs and cats, the calls to bleak Pennine farms to calve cows and castrate pigs, the riding stables with broken-down hacks and a reluctance to pay the bills.

Through Belle Vue I met zoo men from other parts of Britain, and one encounter led to my spending a year and a half at Flamingo Park in Yorkshire where I began to work seriously for the first time with marine mammals. The park's owner, Pentland Hick, sent me around the world on study tours and buying trips, and thus I made friends and clients in the international zoo fraternity. I had a run of luck in always being in the right place at the right time; when the first dart guns were developed, when phencyclidine and M.99, the two most important anaesthetics in the history of wild animal medicine, needed clinical trials, when Windsor Safari Park, the London Dolphinarium, Marineland Côte d'Azur and so many other places opened and looked for veterinary involvement.

Working at Windsor, sometimes travelling down twice within twenty-four hours from my home in the North, brought me into contact with Richard Reed, a free-lance press photographer, and a collection of his pictures of me attending to my exotic patients eventually made the centre pages of the London *Evening Standard*. Because of that I was invited on to the Jack de Manio programme on BBC radio, and John Newth, an editor with the publishers Allen and Unwin, hearing the broadcast, tracked me down with the proposal that I should write my first volume of autobiography, *Zoovet*. 'Zoovet' and its four sequels were eventually turned into three series of drama on BBC television as 'One by One'.

I left Rochdale, divorced (the life of a vet-in-a-suitcase is hard on a marriage) and came to live in Surrey in 1976. By then I had had a partner, Andrew Greenwood, for several years and while he, based in Yorkshire, could cover the North and fly out of Leeds or Manchester, I was better placed for the South and in easy reach of Heathrow and Gatwick.

The jet-vet life itself is one to which I have become addicted. Always on call, always with The Bag packed. A gorilla in Italy today, a dolphin in Spain tomorrow. Then on to Timbuctoo or Toronto. Everyone wants to carry my luggage; exotic places, exotic beasts. Paid to swim with a whale and then relax over Blue Dolphin cocktails, to touch and tend great rarities like pandas and okapis, to eat Thai food this week, Icelandic next, to see a golden monkey in the morning and the Forbidden City in the afternoon, to operate on a circus elephant in Granada and spend the night in the *parador* beside the Alhambra.

Yes, it's all that but . . . Wading in icy water so frequently has taken its toll of my knees, escorting a dolphin or sea elephant on a twelve-hour trip in a cargo jet is chilly, boring, tiring, smelly work. In twenty years, every brief holiday has been interrupted and I've spent fourteen Christmases and as many New Year's Eves away from home, sometimes sitting alone in an airport bar or covered in blood, grease or dirty water beside some desperately ill or injured animal. Going to the toilet so unfailingly causes the telephone to ring that I truly believe there is some sort of circuit between the lavatory seat and British Telecom. There are normally samples of giraffe or whale liver on top of the fish fingers in the deep-freeze and tubes of dolphin blood, ready for pregnancy testing, near the milk in the refrigerator.

The phone begins ringing at five a.m. – it's nine o'clock in Arabia and they've been at work for two hours by then – and it goes on till midnight when my Californian colleagues finally call it a day. Through the post come packets, not always well sealed, of droppings, pus, blood, urine and assorted organs. I've had a raw brain suspected of being rabid arrive in nothing more than brown paper, and other things that smelled appalling after turning into unrecognizable soup in transit.

Nevertheless, I have never picked up any disease from my patients, though some of them have suffered the most bizarre infections, and I collect fewer bites and scratches than most vets in general practice might expect. I've made a lot of money – and happily spent it.

All in all, this *beastly* life is better than anything else I could imagine.

Now read on . . .

1 Hannibal's Animals

Forward, you madman, and hurry across those horrid Alps so
that you may become the delight of schoolboys.

Juvenal, *Satires*

Everyone knows that Hannibal went over the Alps with some
elephants. Full stop. Unless you are a classical scholar, that's
about it. Who Hannibal was and why and how he took to the
high, very high, road, with a herd of jumbos, most of us have
forgotten, if we ever knew.

So when, in 1987, I met Merv Edgecombe for the first time
and he launched at once into an outline of his plans in
the machine-gun-burst style of delivery and mild Yorkshire
accent with which I was going to become very familiar in the
months ahead, I rooted in vain through the attic of my memory
for any dusty recollections of schoolboy lessons on Roman
history forty years before. And found none.

'It's like this, Dave,' (I hate being truncated to 'Dave', but
then, I suppose a 'Merv' would do that naturally). 'What we
want from you is seven weeks. Look after the elephants. Spain
to Italy via France. Ian Botham's going to walk with them
over the Alps. Hundreds of miles. And we don't want any
trouble with the animals.'

I looked at the young man with his close-cropped hair and
confident PR-man's smile. 'Tell us the problems, tell us what
you need,' he continued, 'we'll sort it out.'

'Er . . . well . . .' I began, but then Merv was off again.
'Ian's keen as mustard. Raring to go. And it's all in the best
of causes, to raise cash for the Leukaemia Research Fund.'

Every two or three years someone had contacted me out of
the blue with a similar idea. Once I'd even given a medical
to an elephant at Dudley Zoo, which was supposedly going
on such a march, but nothing had ever come of it.

'If old Hal did it over two thousand years ago, why can't

we?' Merv was still in full flow. 'Including floating them across the River Rhône on rafts!'

'Hold on a minute,' I said. The Alps were one thing, punting five-tonne elephants about on a river that compares for size with the Thames or Rhine was another. 'Are you seriously proposing re-enacting Hannibal's epic journey, yard by yard and mile by mile?'

Merv beamed, 'But of course! Imagine. We'll storm through the gates of Turin, with Beefy Botham on top of the lead elephant! The media will go ape-shit!'

In the year 218 BC there were two great Mediterranean empires, those of Rome and Carthage. Hannibal was a Carthaginian (he would nowadays be an Arab citizen of Tunisia) sworn by his father, Hamilcar Barca, to eternal enmity with Rome, which had recently conquered the Carthaginian territories of Sicily, Sardinia and Corsica. A brilliant general, and only twenty-nine years old, Hannibal already had a string of military successes behind him when he decided to launch a campaign against the heartland of the Roman Empire itself. He would march an army from Carthaginian-occupied Spain east across France and into Italy. His army of around thirty-eight thousand infantry, eight thousand horsemen and thirty-seven elephants would fight their way to the gates of Rome itself – if he could somehow surprise the Romans by entering Italy when and where they least expected it. The way he achieved this is one of the most renowned feats of military history.

'The elephants are the central characters in the walk,' Merv leaned forwards over the table, intense and bright-eyed, the ex-*Daily Mail* reporter on to a scoop. 'They give Ian the glitz that we'll need to keep the media hot to the bitter end.'

I remembered that many years before my friend Dino Terni, the Italian zoo director, had taken one elephant over a small part of Hannibal's route with some English university students. They had encountered no major difficulties – but had only walked for a week or so, all at the elephant's chosen speed. Botham and his fellow walkers would, I knew, set a formidable pace of five or even six miles per hour – for hours on end.

'We set off early each morning,' Merv explained. 'Every town and village we pass through will shower cash for the Fund, there'll be a veritable army of back-up people – mobile kitchen, sports doctor, you name it – and by three o'clock we'll stop and rest up for—'

'Three questions,' I said, interrupting. 'The elephants: how many, where from, and can I have an absolute veto on everything and anything to do with their welfare?'

'Three elephants. From a zoo, we think; it's up to you to advise us. And yes, you can have a veto – what you say goes for the elephants.'

'Zoo elephants won't do,' I replied. 'They can't be relied upon to walk across country, where they'll meet traffic, dogs and people making a noise. It's *got* to be circus elephants. And another thing. No matter what Ian Botham and his friends can do, the elephants can't walk the whole way. For them this can only be a "token walk".'

Mervyn's face dropped. 'What do you mean by that?' he asked.

'No way can they do the fifteen or twenty miles a day that the human walkers will be attempting.'

'But surely . . . in the wild?'

'This isn't "the wild" where they wander browsing through the bush.'

'So what you are saying is . . . ?'

'The elephants aren't even going to *try* keeping up with Botham. That's it, you've given me the veto and I'll exercise it.'

Wild elephants walk at between 2.5 and 3.5 mph, though they can maintain double this speed for several hours if necessary. A charging elephant will reach 25 mph, even though it never runs but rather walks fast. In 218 BC Hannibal's elephants, together with his army, took all summer and autumn to make the great march. The elephant-handlers would have been expected to keep the animals moving along behind the infantry, exhorting them with shouts and prodding them with sticks and spikes. We have records of how far the Carthaginians went in a day, measured in 'stadia', a Roman measurement of length. The trouble is that the scholars aren't exactly sure how long a 'stadium' was: it might have been 177 or 185 metres (190 or 200 yards), and it even seems likely that it was a rather flexible unit of measurement. Hannibal's rate of march was on average eighty stadia per day; probably around fourteen kilometres (say eight miles).

But such historical minutiae didn't trouble me. The Botham elephants would be going for a pleasant stroll every day, the distance never more than a few miles, the exact length dependent on the terrain and weather, and at a speed which would be of their own choosing. What we needed were three good-natured circus elephants, brought up to the roar of the greasepaint, the shouting of clowns and the oompah-oompah of the Big Top band. Accustomed to walking in parade when the circus came to town, they'd be as traffic-proof as police horses and happy among crowds. And the bonus for them, I thought, would be the exercise and Alpine air, for the principal criticism of the anti-circus lobby in regard to elephants is that they don't get enough regular exercise. Botham's expedition would, the way I planned it, be a healthy holiday for a trio of circus jumbos. All we had to do now was find them.

In January 1988, Merv, his director of the expedition, Patsy (he was organizing the walk very much in the same way as one would a large film unit on location) and I flew down to Sicily. A circus, Circo Medrano, was willing to discuss the hire of three elephants. With their winter quarters situated near Verona in northern Italy, the elephants, if we could arrange their participation, would in effect be walking home from Spain.

We found the circus encamped on the harbourside in Palermo and, after we'd introduced ourselves, Ugo, the circus boss, led us to the elephant tent by way of the menagerie of animals that lived all their lives in small travelling cages without even stretching their legs in the ring, a feature of some circuses which cannot be defended. I caught a glimpse of two gorillas languishing in a metal and glass wagon – an unexpected, appalling sight. Gorillas! Highly endangered in their native haunts, but reduced to this among the candy-floss vendors and flashing lights of a tawdry sideshow. Such mini-zoos on wheels continue to exist with standards of design, space and construction which, if applied to a static zoo, would have it closed down within days. It's odd that European governments, including the British, in general seem loath to insist on a tiger in a circus being treated no less well than a tiger in a zoological garden or safari park.

'I wish we could take those gorillas on a walk with Botham through Central Africa,' I said to Merv. He nodded, grim-faced. 'And manage to lose them on the way!' he replied.

In the elephant tent I walked down the line of patient, swaying animals, letting them inspect me with sensitive trunks, sniffing my clothing and giving my pockets a quick frisking for possible sweetmeats.

'These would be the three.' Ugo pointed out the elephants. 'Tali and Dido can't be separated, then there's Batman.' Elephants are like that, they have their special friends. In circuses it has often caused me problems when I have had to keep a sick individual out of the ring or indoors for a few days. It isn't as simple as it sounds. If A stays behind, so must its pal B. Otherwise, all hell can break loose. And on certain occasions I can remember a whole group of elephants refusing, like whales, to be separated from an invalid companion. 'One out, all out' is the motto of the Union of Elephants, and you don't argue with Elephant Solidarity.

Ugo's elephants were of the Indian or Asiatic type; now-adays only two kinds of elephant exist, the African and the Indian. Once there were over three hundred and fifty species of elephant on earth, including a metre-high dwarf form that must have been charming, and a giant that stood almost five metres high, whose fossil remains have been found in Kent.

One of the puzzles about Hannibal's expedition concerns what kind of elephant – African or Indian – he used. The arguments continue in academic circles. He could have obtained either sort; although the African elephant isn't domesticated in its native land nowadays, it is sometimes trained in circuses though it is not in general as easy to handle as the Indian type. Confusingly, Carthaginian coins of 220 BC, just before the expedition, have been found bearing images of African elephants while Indian elephants are depicted on Etrurian coins of 217 BC, the year in which Hannibal conquered that part of northern Italy.

I walked round the three elephants and looked for common weak spots: bent legs, thick legs, swollen joints, cracked toenails, hernias, 'cold' or chronic abscesses. There were none. All three seemed amiable souls. Alert but gentle eyes, salmon-pink gums, plump enough and, most important, passing firm loaf-sized droppings. I poked around in a sample and found the undigested fibre cut small, no sour smell: their teeth and bowels were working fine. (So your offspring wants to be a zoo vet – make him or her understand that a healthy interest in dung in all its forms is more fundamental to a future career than the fact that he/she didn't sleep for a week when the goldfish was found in a terminal state of upside-down floating.)

I then took the elephants' measurements, Taylor the elephant tailor, for any bespoke garments I might decide to order for them. Getting the inside leg of an elephant can be tricky – they tend to be ticklish in the groin.

'Any history of trouble with the three?' I asked Ugo. He shook his head. '*Nada, nada, nada,*' (we were using Spanish as a lingua franca) '*estan en condición perfecta.*' Batman's mighty head nodded as if in agreement and she – for like the other two Batman was a female – squeaked a few contented elephant squeaks. I wondered why she had been given such a ridiculous name.

Back in the circus boss's trailer, negotiations over the fee for the hiring of the three elephants began. Ugo wanted an enormous sum of money, plus so much per day for the keep of the elephants and the handlers who would accompany them. Merv pumped away at his pocket calculator, using the figures I gave him for approximate daily food consumption of an adult elephant: fifty kilos of hay, fifty kilos of fruit and vegetables and two kilos of cereals.

'Anyway, whether we hire them or not they'd have to be fed,' he argued. 'The circus has plenty more elephants, so the show won't suffer. And, damn it all, it *is* for charity.' Bit by bit, Merv beat Ugo down. Eventually, handshakes all round and the elephants were rented at what we considered a fair price. Ugo opened a cold bottle of Berlucchi. Ian Botham's latter-day squadron of war elephants that would lead the campaign for funds to combat leukaemia was enlisted.

Back in England I carefully considered the management of the three elephants during the expedition. Though public support would be enhanced by reports of *human* walkers hobbling bravely on as cramps and fatigue took their toll, the elephants had to have, and be *seen* to have, anything but an arduous journey. I would not permit the smallest blister or slightest degree of tiredness to develop in my charges. The veto on what the elephants could or couldn't do was my key to controlling the situation.

Although I had no opportunity to do a reconnaissance of the intended route, I studied the maps and listed the problems that the elephants, Hannibal's or Botham's, would encounter. Using modern place names, Hannibal's route in 218 BC started in Cartagena, south of Alicante, and went north past Valencia, Barcelona and the Costa Brava. It crossed the Pyrenees and then went along the Mediterranean coast of France by way of Perpignan and Montpellier, and after Nîmes and Avignon reached the River Rhône near Orange. At this point the Carthaginians turned north up the left-hand bank of the Rhône, and were followed by a Roman army that had landed in Marseilles in the hopes of intercepting them. When, however, it seemed that Hannibal was moving in a direction that would lead not to Italy but into the lands of the unruly Gauls, the Romans breathed a sigh of relief and went no further. Seizing the opportunity given by his feint, Hannibal now

crossed the Rhône near Valence, negotiated the Alpine passes
with the help of friendly Gaulish guides, and descended via
the valley of Susa upon the city of the Taurini tribe, Turin.
Astounded, the Romans found Hannibal's army invading the
Po Valley and, after a series of major victories, causing them
to abandon almost the whole of northern Italy.

Our 1988 route followed that of Hannibal at least as far as
the Alpine passes. Which pass the Carthaginian army took
through the mountains is the central enigma of the epic march.
Some historians think they went over the Col de la Traversette,
others the Mont Cenis, and each of five or six possible routes
over the high mountains has its supporters. We were to go
over the Col de Mont Genèvre. My elephants would walk on
metalled roads for most of the way – not for them the icy
boulders of the Alpine cols that I remembered from my
first trekking holidays as a schoolboy just after the war. But
tarmacadam would have its disadvantages too; I would need
to watch their feet like a hawk. Altitude would pose no
problems; our maximum height would be 1,850 metres. Elephants, with their lungs strapped by gristle bands to the inside
of the chest wall, could cope easily with that, and they'd
acclimatize gently in the long coastal approach to the mountains.

Weather, however, was another matter. April in the Hautes
Alpes can be cold, wet and snowy. Elephants, being massive
animals, don't lose heat as easily as say a dog or a rabbit; and
if they're well-fed, able to exercise and acclimatized, adults
stand wet and cold better than you might think for a not very
hairy mammal. Nevertheless, Hannibal lost thirty-six of his
thirty-seven elephants due to severe weather in the year after
crossing the Alps. I could take no chances; the elephants'
normal travelling wagon would have to be always on hand in
case of inclement weather, a tent that could be used as a
'hospital' would need to be carried and each animal would
have a made-to-measure waterproof plastic mac. After much
thought, I dispensed with sets of jumbo-sized leather boots;
I'd used them in the past for single feet to help post-operative

care of septic toes and deformed ankles, but they are tricky things to keep adjusted for animals on the move. If they are thick enough to take the heavy pounding, they can easily pinch and abrade even tough elephant skin.

The next thing was to assemble items for the medical box. What were the possibilities of injury or ailment striking the trio when we were perhaps in some valley where the nearest hamlet was many kilometres away, and veterinary services came in the form of the shepherds' standbys of drenching-bottle, pot of Stockholm tar and sharp penknife? I made a list of kit for most emergencies: some litres of antibiotic injection, cortisone-type drugs for sprains and 'rheumatics' (a term that encompasses a whole range of joint, tendon, ligament and muscle conditions that elephants, like us, can suffer from), sedatives and anaesthetic for minor operations, tubs of creams, ointments and salves for skin afflictions, in an array of colours that would have delighted a medieval apothecary, and, most importantly, brandy.

Brandy for elephants? As I have written elsewhere, old Billy Smart, the circus owner, always insisted on having a bottle of cognac in the medical cupboard. If you find an elephant with a 'cold', a stomach upset after stealing green apples, or a twinge of toothache, something that frequently happens when they change one of their curious, ever-moving teeth, a bottle of brandy will be most gratefully received. Apart from alleviating minor upsets, the major advantage of a bottle of Courvoisier or Hine is that it can be, quickly and simply, *got into the patient.* As a young zoo vet, it didn't take me long to discover that prescribing one pound or half a gallon of this or that nostrum for a peaky pachyderm was worse than useless if it wouldn't swallow it or, like as not, took it into its trunk and then squirted it petulantly all over my head. Elephants have a very acute sense of taste – they'll find a single bitter pill the size of an aspirin hidden in a loaf of bread, and at once return the loaf unceremoniously and often in the most unexpected manner.

Elephants do have a weakness for the grape liquor, however, a fact that doesn't assuage the wrath of the occasional temperance league members who write vitriolic letters to me accusing me of setting dumb animals on the slippery path. These good folk should watch elephants and baboons in Africa seeking out and gorging on the overripe, alcohol-loaded fruit of the miracle tree at the right time of year. Now those are really *wild* parties!

So, through the good offices of the landlord of my local pub, the Half Moon, I arranged for the distillers to donate a crate of Rémy Martin to the walk, principally for the medical treatment of elephants.

Just before the big press conference held at the Oval to announce details of the walk, I noticed a brief report in the *Veterinary Record* – African horse sickness, a virulent midge – or mosquito-borne virus disease, had broken out in Spain, probably due to the importation of a number of infected zebras. Elephants aren't susceptible to the disease, but the movement of animals across Spanish borders might be restricted as a consequence of the epidemic. I rang Merv and asked him to check on the situation with the Spanish and, more importantly, the French authorities. I met Ian and Kathy Botham for the first time just before the conference started, and found the cricketer and his wife to be down-to-earth characters, devoid of sports-star self-importance and deeply committed to the anti-leukaemia campaign. They were as anxious as I was to ensure that the elephants would come first at all times.

Then, half an hour before Ian spoke to the crowd of journalists, Merv came up to me. 'We are in the cow-pat as far as the full seven-week expedition is concerned,' he told me. 'The French aren't permitting *any* entry of horses or other big livestock coming from Spain. They say the stiuation may change if the Spaniards get the epidemic quickly under control, but there are no guarantees of that.' Leaving the elephants behind, trapped in Spain, was something we couldn't contemplate. Merv went into a series of brief and frantic meetings with his associates, with the Bothams, with the major sponsor, a finance company, and with Yorkshire Television who were to cover the whole event. It was decided to lop the Spanish section off the walk; we would start instead at Perpignan in France – the expedition would in consequence last for only one month. It was a blow, but not a critical one. A month with daily media coverage could still raise a lot of money for the cause; and though Yorkshire Television at once cancelled their plans to send a film crew along with us, their place was taken by Television South. I was delighted to hear that their team would be led by David Pick, an old friend through whom, twelve years before, I had begun my association with the Southampton-based television company.

Two days before the start of the walk I arrived in Perpignan and met most of the people who would be taking part. Besides the Bothams there was a core of about a dozen people, including Greg Richie, the Australian cricketer, who were planning to walk the whole way. Around twice that number were hoping to manage various proportions of the distance. There were three television crews and a gaggle of reporters in hire cars who would follow in comfort. Then there was a large back-up team of 'fixers', messengers, drivers and caterers (many of them volunteers who had accompanied Ian on previous charity walks); the handful of Italian circus men looking after the elephants; Steve Carroll, the medical officer, who was an expert in the treatment of sports injuries; Wolfgang Zeuner, a historian and Hannibal specialist, who for years had planned such an expedition; and Rex Shayler, who was both walker and electronics wizard. It was Rex who had designed and built the physiology-monitoring equipment. He had come up with the idea of connecting an ingenious little box of tricks, which the elephants would carry on a light harness, to small adhesive patches stuck on their skin. Information on the animal's pulse, respiration and – it was claimed – other bodily functions would be transmitted by a built-in radio to a receiver-recorder in a vehicle travelling along slowly behind the elephants. There was even an alarm with flashing red light if any animal showed signs of stress.

For my part I was more than willing to try out the monitoring equipment, but I had doubts as to whether it would work on the move. As for the alarm – great, but I had no intention of allowing the elephants even to get out of puff, as we say in Lancashire, let alone suffer stress. My eyes and ears, and occasionally my stethoscope, are the instruments I trust most in assessing an elephant's health and happiness.

Day One of the walk dawned cold and showery, with a cloudy sky the colour of an elephant's back. A lively breeze blew through the old city gate as everyone assembled at the start. The elephants arrived in their wagons at eight o'clock and I checked them over before Rex began fitting them up with the monitors and harness. Around us things were not proceeding smoothly; there were parking problems, altercations between stewards and pushy photographers and the difficulties of setting banners in the wind. Reporters stood grumpily puffing through chilly hands, policemen blew whistles as if on impulse, children in traditional Provençal costume strained to hear the music above the din as they danced pale-faced, and the French populace, gloomily on their way to work, regarded the little crowd of short-panted, silly-hatted Englishmen and three elephants with blank incomprehension and hurried by. Merv was standing swearing; he had just been informed that in France it was forbidden to collect money as the walk went along. Such 'begging', even for charity, was illegal.

Suddenly Botham, who had been talking with friends in the centre of the crowd, set off through the gate at a brisk pace. No gun, no fanfare. It just happened. These unexpected starts, when Ian simply said 'I'm off', were to be routine occurrences. Chaos ensued. Botham, with the knot of serious walkers in tow, burst out of the crowd. 'Come on, get the elephants on the move!' I shouted to Davio, the head elephant-man. He didn't react. I repeated it in Spanish: '*Vamonos!*' He shouted it in Italian to his team, and at last the three elephants got under way.

Photographers, dancers, policemen, distributors of bacon

rolls and innocent passers-by, all reeled out of the way as Tali, Dido and Batman swept forward in line astern, trumpeting gaily. Hurrying behind the hind legs of the third elephant, I wondered what it was like when Hannibal's army had set out after camping overnight near here over two millennia ago. Similar noisy confusion I supposed. Similar people, too. We know there was a chief army doctor, Synhalus, and an army chaplain with the we hope inappropriate name of Bogus. Whether there was a Carthaginian equivalent of me, we don't know.

The elephants were walking fast to keep up with Botham's group but, even so, they were falling behind as we went through the centre of Perpignan. Davio shouted encouragement to the animals to keep them at full speed, and their legs slapped hard against the canvas webbing of the monitor harness which had been loosely assembled around the buttocks to prevent chafing. After the first three hundred metres of the seven-hundred-kilometre journey, bits of Rex's harness, wires, adhesive patches, buckles and plastic battery pouches littered the road – and we couldn't stop to pick them up. So much for the monitoring programme. We never used it again.

Trotting along behind Batman, and skipping occasionally to avoid droppings that thudded in my path, I quickly realized that the elephants' speed had to be cut back sharply. At this pace they would soon tire; like me they were out of condition. Circus life is too sedentary. 'Slow them down, let them take their time,' I shouted to Davio.

'But, doctor, the walkers are already half a kilometre in front.'

'No matter. We start as we shall go on. The elephants pick the speed.' Batman and Co. slowed to an effortless amble.

My plan for a 'token walk' was the only way; if the weather was reasonable and the going not too tough, we would set off with the walkers each morning, do a kilometre or two at our own pace, load up the elephants and drive them on to a point not far from the next big village, where they could enjoy themselves in a field or patch of woodland. When the walkers eventually caught up, the animals would lead them through the streets and then travel on by vehicle again until just short of the day's finishing line, where they would again roam free until the sore and sweating Botham came into sight. Using this system the elephants walked on average eight or nine kilometres of the route each day, while the humans tramped on four times as far non-stop, snatching drinks and sandwiches as they went. The elephants got abundant exercise, never became tired and were always in the right place to draw crowds and be presented to Monsieur le Maire. In France and Italy, where few people have even seen a cricket bat, let alone heard of Botham, Batman and her friends were the key to our publicity, for the world over elephants are wondrous beasts, more popular with people than any other species.

The showers stopped and we soon found ourselves outside the city, walking along a dry, level road. We came to a field where three horses ran excitedly to the fence, ears pricked and tails aloft, to watch our progress. The elephants didn't like the look of them. They began to trumpet petulantly and passed them with their bodies skewed crab fashion, and their shiny eyes glaring. 'They detest horses,' hollered Davio. I wondered how they managed with the equestrian acts that they must surely meet in the circus. From then on I asked people at the head of the march to pass the word back if they saw any equines along the route – elephants running amok in the French countryside was something best avoided. One of the advantages of Hannibal's battle elephants was their terrorizing effect on the horses of opposing cavalry. Later, the Romans were to bring elephants with their armies to fight against the Britons and when these animals, armoured and carrying towers holding archers and sling-throwers, crossed the Thames in the battle for Londinium (London), they caused a panicked scattering of the British cavalry.

We had been walking for about forty-five minutes, with me running round the elephant procession from time to time to check their gait, when I noticed a slight change in the style of movement of Batman's right foreleg. She was swinging it outwards an inch or two just before it touched the ground. I observed it from all angles as she walked. It was barely perceptible, she wasn't really limping but . . . After a further ten minutes had passed, I was certain that the outward swing was more pronounced and Davio, who knew her far better than I did, agreed when I pointed it out to him. Disaster! Not three miles out on the first day and walking on the flat on smooth tarmac, Batman had gone lame.

I gave the order to turn off into the car-park of a roadside motel, and there inspected the elephant's limb from toe-nails up to shoulder. There was heat and a little tenderness around the elbow joint. The joint capsule was inflamed – for no apparent reason. I went to the medical box, and made up an injection of fast-acting corticosteroid. Five minutes later, surrounded by the reporters and photographers who seemed gratified at this early augury of an action-packed trip, I delivered the official medical bulletin on Batman – she would ride in the wagon for the next couple of days while I continued treatment. If she became completely sound, she then could rejoin the walk. If she didn't – at that precise moment Batman urinated and the torrent poured over my feet. I joined in the general laughter, but at the back of my mind something niggled. Why had Batman broken down so quickly?

The next day, only two elephants took to the road and I stayed behind for a while to examine Batman and give more of the anti-flammatory injection. She had improved, but was still throwing the leg. My medical box was carried in the cab of the elephant wagon and, while I was in there routing about for disposable quarter-pint syringes and needles, I noticed a cardboard box bearing a medical label projecting from beneath the driver's seat. It wasn't any of my stock; I pulled it out to see what it was. The box was filled with dozens of bottles of corticosteroid injection, and there were needles and syringes too. Altogether there were enough drugs to have treated all of Hannibal's army if every soldier had got javelin-hurler's kneecap, sword-wielder's wrist, or whatever their ancient occupational diseases were. The driver of the elephant wagon was outside and I went to buttonhole him. Though I don't speak any more Italian than is needed to distinguish my Barolo from my Bardolino, he understood my question. Waving one of the bottles of injection I said '*La medicina – perchè?*'

'*Oh. E per Batman.*'

'*Batman frequentemente piccoli problemi con—*' I slapped my elbow.

'Si, si. *Frequentemente. Ma iniezione sempre funzionanno molto bene!*'

So that was it. The circus carried the drug routinely for Batman's recurring 'little problem'. When she went lame she'd be given a shot without benefit of veterinarian, and in a few days no doubt be sound enough, at least for the public to see nothing amiss. Her elbow joint wasn't deformed or thickened, but there was obviously a long-standing weakness, arising perhaps from a sprain or other injury years before. And the circus hadn't said a thing about it to us when contracting to send Batman with Botham on the Long March to Turin.

Compared with many cases of lameness that I'd had to deal with in elephants over the years, Batman's sore elbow was insignificant. But unless she was one hundred per cent sound, and likely to remain so, I couldn't return her to the walk with all its attendant publicity. Already, back in England, some of the anti-zoo and circus folk, before taking the trouble to find out the facts, had been shrilling about how the lameness of Batman was what they had predicted if elephants were forced to climb mountain peaks. After two more days on the corticosteroid, Batman was within a whisker of normal. Only an expert could detect the faint swing of the leg that remained. I made the decision – Batman should not continue with the walk, and I wasn't prepared to have her in the elephant wagon for most of the day. She would go back to the circus for rest among her friends, and I would visit her there.

We continued through Provence by way of Narbonne and

Béziers. From time to time celebrities would join us for a day or two to walk, and occasionally to ride on the elephants. They included the rock guitarist Eric Clapton, Eddie 'The Eagle' Edwards of ski-ing failure fame, and some well-known sportsmen and women. The route was still over mainly flat country. We started and finished each day in a village or small town and, although the French people seemed on the whole rather apathetic towards us, the elephants' carefree stealing of fruit, vegetables and confectioneries as we went by shops and markets where these wares were on display outside was tolerated amiably. If Tali or Dido lifted an onion or two from a tray, the shopkeeper would invariably rush out to offer the lot. I had to keep an eye on such free-loading. The effect of elephants gorging themselves had occupied me so many times in the past – the consequent cataract of diarrhoea and miserable colics. On chilly mornings when I thought my charges were rather 'peaky', I gave them a slug of half a bottle of cognac, pouring it into the end of their trunks which they willingly curled up into a U-shaped cup that was then thrust into their mouths and sucked dry with evident delight.

As the days passed the elephants' condition, like that of the humans, steadily improved. The fresh air, ever-changing scenery and exercise did them a power of good, and I noticed that they spontaneously increased their rate of march. Once Batman left us the weather remained dry, cool and often sunny for the rest of the journey through France. Wherever possible I scouted ahead in a car to find something like a mud-wallow, thicket or shallow pool in which the elephants could enjoy themselves. Although Botham wouldn't stop for anybody or anything when walking – even people who flew in to present cheques to him had to do it 'on the hoof' – he was always willing to make a diversion from the route to go with the animals through some bit of countryside that gave them special pleasure. At Cap d'Agde they paddled in the sea, and outside Montpellier they spent a morning wandering happily in a vineyard where the vine stocks were low and gnarled at that time of the year, though the elephants were so delicate in placing their feet that they didn't damage a single plant. Always contented, they regularly made the pleasing loud purring noise that elephants make when all is right with the world. The animals revelled in the new sights, sounds and smells, the wayside herbs to be sampled and the constant trickle of humans bearing edible gifts.

And there were other things, like the day two Englishmen, one a vet I knew, arrived from an organization called Zoo Check 'to investigate' us. I don't imagine they would have flown out to check on any of the thousand and one elephants travelling with Continental circuses, but with us there was the possibility of poaching some of Botham's publicity. We had, from the beginning, welcomed visits from anyone from animal welfare organizations, and indeed the French equival-ent of the RSPCA gave the Walk a donation after sending a representative to see how the animals were being treated. The Zoo Check couple seemed bent on 'exposing' something or other, for they skulked about, ran away from reporters in the most ridiculous fashion and didn't turn up for a press conference to which they were invited. The problem for them, I suppose, was that the elephants were patently being well cared for, and if one complains about circus elephants not getting enough exercise, it is difficult then to argue that they shouldn't go on easy country walkabouts.

When Hannibal came to the River Rhône he faced several problems – a Roman army on his tail, hostile tribesmen on the opposite bank and the need to get his elephants across the wide expanse of water. In 1988 it was only the last task which concerned us.

Hannibal built rafts, moored them securely to the bank and covered them with sods of earth to make them appear like projections of the dry land. Elephants are understandably frightened of ground that gives under foot, and normally refuse to put their weight on to anything that wobbles in the slightest. The last elephant to leave Belle Vue Zoo in Manchester died because of a ramp that she didn't want to climb after feeling the wood give a little. Hannibal's engineers apparently did an excellent job, for all the elephants boarded the rafts which were then cast off and towed or punted across the river. Some elephants, panicking, upset their rafts and men and animals fell into the water. We don't know whether any men perished but none of the elephants were drowned, for they were in shallow water and continued the crossing by walking on the river bottom with their trunks held up above the surface. Elephants invented snorkels many thousands of years before men first went diving!

Merv and his team had arranged for British Army and French Foreign Legion men to provide us with army rafts for our re-enactment of the Rhône crossing. I was apprehensive about the scheme and, not having seen any of the proposed equipment, worried that it, too, might easily be destabilized and perhaps capsized by three five-tonne giants suddenly becoming nervous and very literally rocking the boat. Fortunately for me and the elephants, though not for the television crews and press photographers, I was not called upon to decide whether to risk the raft crossing. A few days before we reached Orange on the Rhône, the Army pulled out of the operation and we subsequently crossed the river in safe, if unspectacular fashion, by way of the road bridge.

A week after Batman had left us, Merv and I drove down to Toulon where the circus was pitched for a couple of weeks. We took with us several one-pound bags of sugar cubes, the elephant equivalent of grapes for the human hospital patient. I found the elephant to be walking sound once more, with no sign of anything amiss with the elbow. But much as I loved the friendly animal, I had lost trust in the joint and turned down Ugo's offer to return her to the Walk. During the rest of the Walk, apart from one instance when Tali stood on the prong of a pitchfork and suffered a small penetrating wound of the sole of one foot, I didn't have any accidents or outbreaks of disease in my couple of patients. By contrast, Steve, the medical officer, was constantly at work with giant blisters, sprains, foot infections, toe-nail removals and even a fracture of the shin caused by excessive walking – he was a magician whose techniques could, I swear, have got a man with no legs on the march again.

In Nîmes there are several important, well-preserved Roman ruins, including the amphitheatre and a temple, the Maison Carrée. The elephants were filmed by TVS making an impressive entrance into the arena of the amphitheatre; then, rashly, I agreed to them going up the steps of the Maison Carrée to stand under the great portico of the building. The flight of steep, shallow, stone steps was easily negotiated by the animals *going up*, but to my dismay it began to rain when they were both being filmed at the top. Their feet were broader than the depth of a step and their weight would be tipped forwards coming down the smooth stone, which had almost immediately become slippery. I realized that the slightest mistake would result in a horrendous fall. Fractured legs usually mean dead elephants. What a fool I'd been! My stomach turned to ice.

Some of the television crew were standing nearby. 'Quick!' I shouted. 'Get any dirt or gravel you can find – scratch it up with *anything* and sprinkle it on the steps.' We all began searching for patches of bare earth. A camera assistant used his clapper-board to scoop soil, a researcher raked at the ground with the end of a microphone pole. I told Davio to keep the elephants under the portico until we had gritted the staircase as well as we could. It didn't look much, but perhaps it would help.

The rain slackened to a steady drizzle. When we were ready, I decided to bring the elephants down backwards. That way they would perhaps fall into the steps and slide down on their bellies if they lost their foothold. The disadvantage was that they couldn't see where they were going and had to feel their way blind, aided only by the gentle encouragement of Davio, murmuring to them in the pidgin German that is the common language of circus elephants.

First was Tali. Very, very slowly, tentatively searching and tapping for the step with her sensitive toe-tip, she found a

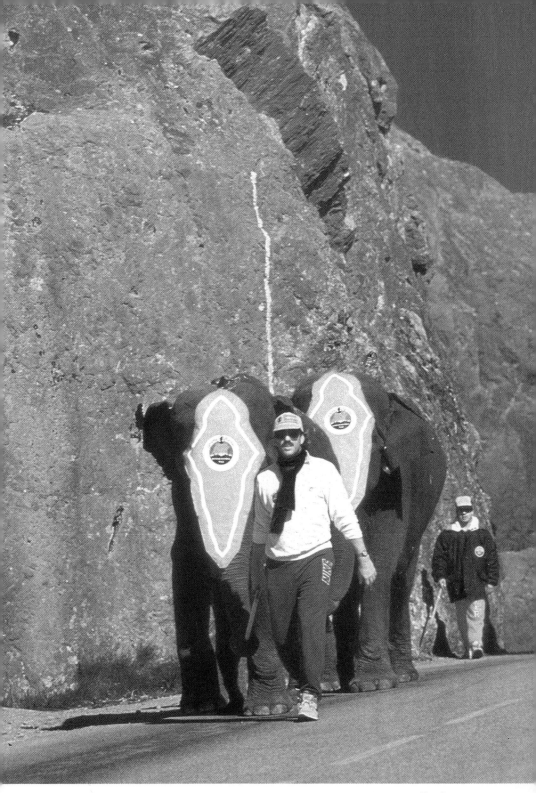

Unlike the elephants on the Hannibal walk, Ian Botham walked every inch of the way! (*Rex Features*)

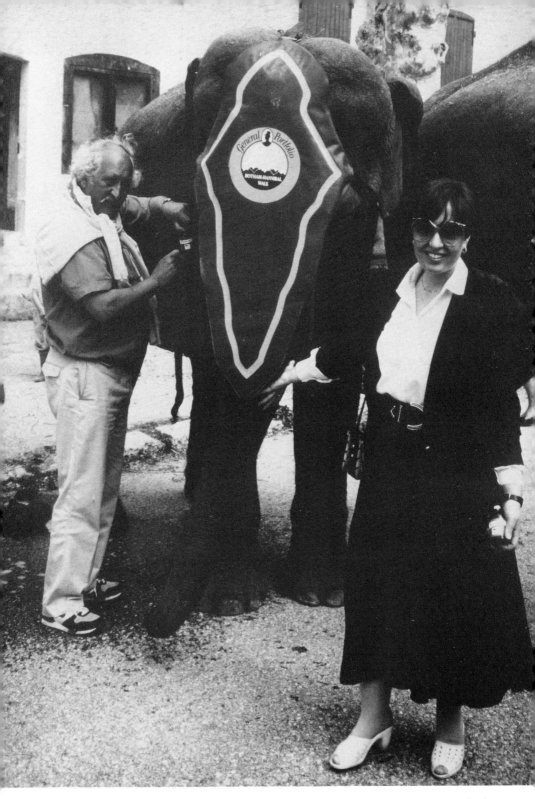

'Batman' receives an injection after being pulled out of the Hannibal walk near Perpignan. (*Graham Morris*)

hold for the front half of her hind foot, carefully tilted her weight on to it, balanced and then inched back a forefoot. It was an awesome sight. The great grey bottom of the elephant poised over the steep drop and the patient, methodical, snail's pace of the limb movement. The minutes passed. David Pick, the producer, was ashen-faced and leaned against a pillar, unable to watch, while I felt like vomiting. But the enormous grey bulk of the elephant was steadily descending. We were witnessing a rare demonstration of the measured control of power. I, a stupid human, had got them up there and now these great animals were getting themselves down by sheer intelligence, concentration and agility. After what seemed a year Tali stood before me on level ground, snuffling in my pockets for sugar, as calm as a cucumber and looking as unconcerned about her mastery of the heights as if she were a chamois rather than an elephant.

Now it was Dido's turn. We could still have a tragedy on our hands. But Dido proved as nimble a performer as her companion and used the same ungainly-looking but successful back-end-first technique. When at last she was safely down we cheered for all we were worth, and then David and I slunk off to the nearest bar for large brandies to steady our nerves. I'll never forget my mistake at the Maison Carrée.

With the country becoming more hilly as we approached the Alps, we were keeping to the valleys and there was little in the way of gradient to trouble the elephants. When the elephants walked, I walked, when they relaxed on an Alpine meadow with Botham and the 'serious' walkers panting towards them ten kilometres back, I had time to explore the wayside churches and sample the wines and cheeses of Languedoc. Only two severe climbs awaited the walkers, the Col de Cabre and the Col de Mont Genèvre, and I made a reconnaissance of these high passes by car and decided that the elephants would do no more than a few hundred metres on each of them, and none at all if the weather was bad. Each day I inspected the elephants and had been pleased to note that by the time we reached Pont de Quart their feet were in perfect condition. Circus elephants frequently develop overgrown soles due to having relatively little exercise. The horny pads become very thickened and sometimes under-run by smelly, rotten erosions which need prompt attention. Chiropody, in the shape of a vet or blacksmith paring away the excess sole and cleaning out the decaying patches, is an essential routine for elephants who don't do plenty of walking. And elephants won't always obligingly lift up their feet like some world-weary pony to let you chisel and chop away, painless though it is. There are some circus-trained elephants who will lie down on one side on command, and let me work with my collection of files, pincers and knives, but most of the others need sedatives or even anaesthetics so that I can work without being kicked, belaboured by the trunk or simply sat upon.

As we entered the final week of the walk, however, I saw that our elephants' feet had been not only pared down and cleaned by the walking on asphalted roads, but that there was now the first sign of the beautifully smooth white soles continuing to be thinned by contact with the sharp granite particles in the asphalt. The animals were walking fast and enthusiastically but, even with the few kilometres they were doing each day, there was a risk that before long I might be faced with tender feet. At once I informed everybody that from there on the elephants would walk only one or two kilometres a day and spend the rest of the time out at grass or as guests of honour at the civic receptions.

Despite fears (and secret hopes, I suspect, on the part of the media) that the climb over the Cols might trigger cardiovascular crises in one or two of the walkers, they all made it – and quicker than anticipated. The weeks of walking had made everyone, including the elephants and me, much fitter; and now the animals, still picking their own speed, could almost keep up with Botham and the leaders whenever they set off together. Bitter winds and rain confined the elephants to their wagon when we traversed the Col de Cabre, but on the Mont Genèvre we would cross the French–Italian border and we'd have only two days' journey downhill to Turin still ahead of us. I decided to let the elephants have their final stroll in the high mountains. It was cold and foggy and snow lay on the ground as Tali and Dido solemnly marched over the border, to be greeted by a large and happy crowd of people in traditional costume. There were soldiers and musicians straight out of Italian opera, carnival figures and, yes, an *Italian* cricket team from Turin – all wreathed in the grey and clammy mist. To the blare of a brass band and the excited clapping and chatter of the crowd, we began the descent into Italy, led by the colourful throng. The elephants must have felt they were back in the grandest of circus parades.

The entry into the busy metropolis with its teeming traffic was something of an anti-climax. Where Hannibal's army had swept in and conquered the stronghold of the Taurini, we battled to keep the walkers from being split up and run over by the Italian motorists, and walked with a protective cordon around the elephants to stop children darting into their path and getting injured. At last, after twenty-one days' journey, Ian and Kathy Botham, and the rest of the gallant band who had legged it every inch of the way, stood with the elephants in the great Piazza Castello before the town hall.

While Botham and the others attended a civic reception in their honour, I said farewell to the elephants, for the wagon was ready to take them straight back to the circus. The remaining sugar lumps were dispensed and, for the last time, their trunk tips delicately rippled through my hair and inside my jacket. Like Hannibal, we hadn't lost an elephant – though he'd had twelve times as many. Apart from Botham's magnificent effort in raising so much cash for a vitally import- ant cause, the walk had also given something valuable to the gentle elephants – a once-in-a-lifetime taste, however small, of freedom. Wouldn't it be great if every circus elephant was entitled to an Alpine holiday from time to time?

2 Running After Rhino

But you'll never become a rhinoceros, really you won't . . . you
haven't got the vocation.

Eugène Ionesco, *Rhinoceros*

So the *Arabian Nights* got it wrong. It was clearly stated that
I should see two human figures when I had finished cutting.
Try as I might, I couldn't make them out.

This was in 1960 and, as a young vet exploring the still
largely unknown realms of zoological medicine, I was in the
dispensary cum clinic cum head keeper's sanctum attached
to the Victorian-built elephant house at Belle Vue in Manchester. After months of effort we had finally lost the battle to keep
the old female rhinoceros alive. She had been an irascible and
uncooperative patient right to the end, when her weight had
plummeted so that she was little more than bones clothed in
iron-hard hide. The weight loss had been accompanied by the
intermittent appearance of blood in her urine. My diagnosis,
based on no experience and with the few colleagues in London
and Chester Zoos who'd ever been called to see any sort of
sick rhinoceros unable to suggest anything better, was chronic
kidney disease.

Safe, easily administered sedatives for such formidable animals had yet to be developed so sampling blood for analysis
from an ear vein was impossible, although on one occasion,
Matt Kelly, the well-known Irish head keeper and Mancunian
'character' did get some blood from her by quick thinking.

I'd tried everything by way of medication from streptomycin
injected after putting her in a massive steel handling crate, or
crush, each day and literally hammering the biggest hypodermic needle I could find into her buttocks, to pints of cider
vinegar poured into her drinking water. This was at the
suggestion of my father; at the time cider vinegar and honey
was in vogue as a popular panacea, and he swore it had done

simultaneous wonders for his arthriticky knees, catarrh and haemorrhoids. Certainly I had the impression that the rhino improved for a while with the cider vinegar, something that hadn't happened with anything else. But there was the difficulty in those days of having to use the metal crush on a regular basis. It was the only way of giving injections, but the animal detested the contraption and crashed about in it irritably, making the six-inch steel posts tremble and dust shower down from the roof timbers. In the process she abraded the skin over her ridged face and buttocks, and though it wasn't serious and she was unaware of the superficial lacerations, they had to be treated with antiseptic creams, for rhino skin is very prone to infection, and the thinner she became, the more protuberances there were revealed that could be damaged. That meant more use of the crush and so on – a vicious circle.

One night, Matt phoned me to say that he'd obtained the blood sample from the rhino which I had for so long impotently desired.

'Me bhoy, oi've got a bit of the claret for ye. Will it be enough for your experimentin'?' Matt in those days was the terror of young vets like me. A man of great charm and charisma, he was one of the best of the 'old school' of zoo men. Long on experience, expert and skilful when it came to enticing a weakly gazelle calf to drink or an elephant to open its mouth, they had little time for tyros like me – full of book-learning and new-fangled nonsense, but unacquainted with the subtle ways of handling delicate or fierce cold-blooded or hot-tempered exotica. Matt was an artist – he knew how to catch a conscious leopard safely by the tail, the herbs that could tempt a listless antelope to eat, the way to hypnotize a crocodile and the knack of recapturing an escaped hummingbird by attracting it with a bright flower. He understood and was greatly loved by chimpanzees and elephants, he had brought back a great collection of hoofed animals by boat from Africa to Manchester single-handed, and he could talk the hind leg off a donkey. I learned a great deal from him;

and eventually, grudgingly, in the years to come he was to learn something from me and what he called 'cesstatious science', whatever that meant.

So my mentor had got some blood from the rhino. How, I wondered. What arcane bit of Irish ingenuity had he demonstrated yet again? But it was simple enough. He explained that the rhino had lunged at him as he was perched on the side of the crush smearing ointment on her, and she had nicked her lip. The small wound dripped slowly, and he had dashed to the dispensary for a heparin tube of the sort he'd seen me use to collect blood from more easily sampled animals. He cautiously put an arm through the bars of the crush, risking having it pulped, and, taking care not to touch the animal, gathered six or seven drops before it stopped. It was enough to do a few basic tests. The rhino proved to be profoundly anæmic and the anæmia was of the haemolytic kind – the red blood cells were being destroyed within the circulation system by something, in a similar way to what happens in severe malaria of human beings. We still don't know the true cause, or causes, of this syndrome, which I have seen several times since then in rhinos, but I believe it is generally a form of Weil's disease, the dreaded rat-borne disease which infected miners in the old days and, more recently, has been suffered by water-skiers using for their sport flooded gravel pits where rodents lurk and contaminate the water.

When the Belle Vue rhino died, Matt was very keen that I should saw off the animal's horn. It was well shaped and about thirty centimetres (a foot or so) long. I was naive in those days.

'What do you want it for?' I asked the head keeper.

'Well, as a souvenir, ye know. She was an old friend,' he replied.

'What will you do with it?'

'Ohh, polish it, mount it or somethin'.'

'It's the first rhino horn I've had the opportunity to examine in detail. I was hoping to cut it, to look at its structure in detail – it's not horn you know, it's really just tightly compacted hair.'

Matt's face took on the sour 'more scientific malarkey' look that I was getting to know well, and he clicked his teeth. After a long pause he said, 'Well, go ahead then and cut it, if ye must. One cut, moind. Don't chop the whole bejasus to smithereens!'

'If I cut it in two, it'll make two souvenirs. Perhaps I could have one.'

'Err, well . . . erm . . . no, come to think of it, oi'll give half to my friend in Tib Street.'

'Tib Street?'

Sounding now rather exasperated, he said 'Yes. I've a friend down there who swears boi rhinoceros horn for headaches, nose bleeds and all manner o' things.'

'What on earth does he do with the horn – stew it?'

'Oh, I don't know. But he says it's done a world of good for his headaches – the only thing for migraine. *Doctors* aren't much use, ye know,' he added with emphasis.

There are so many legends about rhinoceros horn. Which is where the *Arabian Nights* come in. In the second voyage of Sinbad the Sailor, it is related that, if a rhino horn is cut in two lengthways, 'several white lines will be seen representing human figures'. I didn't see the lines when I sawed that first horn in front of Matt, and I haven't seen them since in any of the dozens of horns I've had to remove for surgical reasons.

Another fable, and one long believed, was that if a suspect liquid were put into a cup made of rhino horn, it would effervesce if it were poisonous. But the best-known bit of nonsense, and the one with appalling consequences for rhinos as a species, is the belief that rhino horn is a powerful medicine and aphrodisiac. In the Far East there is an enormous demand for rhinoceros horn as an ingredient of potions used in traditional medicine. The aphrodisiac qualities of the stuff are not, as we tend to think in the West, the main attraction, but rather its reputation in treating conditions of the head and nose. I suppose the reasoning goes that, growing where it does, the horn must be a repository of all that is strong and powerful in that part of the body.

Thirty years ago, at the time of that first rhino death in Belle Vue, there was little attention paid by the world in general to such things as rhino poaching and its connection to a trade in horns. When Matt presented me with a bottle of whisky a week later – a gift, he said, from his friend Mr Cheung in Tib Street as thanks for the present of some horn (actually I think Matt sold him both halves) which was certain to alleviate his bothersome migraine – I didn't give it much thought; it was another of Matt's perks, like rendering down the fat of a bear I'd post-mortemed to sell as a much-vaunted Lancashire cure for rheumatism, or collecting the cast tail feathers of the peacocks that wandered round the grounds for Manchester florists, who used them in flower arranging.

At that time there were perhaps seventy-five thousand black rhino in Africa. Now their numbers are down to around four thousand. In the 1970s, and even more in the 1980s, we became belatedly aware of what was happening to the rhino in Africa. Poachers with powerful automatic weapons continue to slaughter the animals, drawn by the riches that can be theirs for selling horns to the Far East for the medicine makers and to North Yemen in Arabia for carving into traditional 'jambia' dagger handles. One big horn can fetch up to £50,000!

Sometimes I have to amputate a rhino horn where it has been damaged by fighting, or has grown in a curve that threatens to press into the flesh of the face. What am I to do with these lumps of wood-like material, each weighing four or five kilos? Firstly, it must be said that in this country they could be sold easily for export to Hong Kong, Macao or Taiwan by devious routes. From time to time, I get calls from people, not always with oriental accents, asking me to bear them in mind when I come across rhino horn disconnected from its rightful owner. These folk also show an intense interest in genitalia – of tigers, lions, sea lions and deer – apparently imagining that my week is spent gelding these exotic creatures rather than encouraging them to reproduce. And the prices they suggest for, say a deep-frozen tiger penis or pair of leopard testicles, are staggering – enough to make any big cat that overheard and understood such telephonic absurdities clutch his groin and run. Secondly, my partner Andrew and I would never dream of selling rhino horn or the private parts of other beasts, for the major reason that, although an animal which has died in the zoo or safari park of natural causes has no further need of these appendages, and though no poaching or other cruelty would be involved, it would contribute to the trade in these things, helping, if only in a small way, its survival and prosperity. That's the last thing we want.

But of course rhinos, like humans and other animals, continue to die – if only from old age – from time to time. More than once, when I have performed a post-mortem on a rhinoceros, someone has then sneaked in and removed a horn while I was showering or having a meal with the zoo director. When, in 1988, I sawed off the damaged horn of a white rhino at Windsor Safari Park, an attempt was made to steal the 'trophy' from the office of my friend Terry Nutkins, where I had left it on the shelf. I am now of the opinion that the best thing for these accursed protuberances is to burn them as soon as they are cut off.

It was June 1987. Standing on the white-dust road beneath an implacable mid-afternoon sun, just outside the town of Massa, north of Pisa, the Italian soldier – a member of the corps who serve as police – hitched the strap of his sub-machine gun over the left-hand shoulder of his smart but oppressive dark-blue uniform. Bees hummed over the yellowing verges. The occasional car, open-windowed with radio blaring full volume, passed by. He could smell nothing but dust and hot air. The *caribiniere* was in a post-prandial mood. Two hours to go to the end of the shift and lunch, taken as usual in Giuseppe's, still lingered agreeably in his stomach – the *carpaccio*, the *linguini ai funghi* and the Tuscan wine. Tomorrow would be his saint's day, Lorenzo di Brindisi, he had the day off and Milano were playing football on television.

Life was *molto bene* round these parts. No mafiosi like Palermo or Calabria, no Red Brigade terrorists, none of the frenzied crush of Roma. Nothing much in fact. *Molto bene*. Which suited him and his heavily pregnant wife down to the ground. The *carabiniere* looked down the road to his right where it made a bend over the railway crossing. *Madonna!* Walking towards him was a rhinoceros. No mistake – he'd seen one once at the zoo in Torino and others on television films. Grey against the white dust, horn pointed menacingly straight at him, the great beast was lumbering steadily in his direction.

Rhinoceroses, as the *carabiniere* knew for certain, are not members of the native Italian fauna. There are a few wolves and brown bears in places, water buffalo have been domesticated and can be seen working on farms, there are wild boar, vultures, eagles, marmots and chamois in the Alpine regions and three kinds of venomous viper, but since prehistoric times there haven't been any Italian rhinos. But here it was, strolling along like a cow going home for milking. No zoo or safari park for miles around. It couldn't be an escaper, surely. He didn't feel ill, and the amount of wine he'd drunk at lunch was no more than his accustomed two *bicchieri*. The *carabiniere* unslung his machine-gun and looked round, heart thumping, for somewhere to hide. This fierce beast that had materialized out of the Romagnan soil could be a man-eater!

Fifty yards up the road, away from the rhinoceros, was the edge of a vineyard. He ran for all he was worth, jumped down the shallow bank and crashed through the nearest row of leafy vines. Turning, he fell to a crouch, and peered through the foliage. *Miracoloso*, the monster wasn't following him! It was continuing to walk sedately along the road and would soon be level with him.

At that moment he heard voices. A group of men came into view; they were about a hundred metres behind the rhinoceros and some were running. There were at least ten of them, several carried coils of rope and they were led by, *madonna*, two of the local policemen who were chattering furiously and waving their pistols in the air.

The rhino's name was Tommy. The last time I'd seen him in the flesh was when he was a two-year-old; he'd been born at Longleat Safari Park and I'd gone there at the request of an Italian zoo-dealer to give the animal a clean bill of health. Like most of the white rhinos born in safari parks (and Longleat's breeding record in this respect has contributed as much as any to the successful saving of this species from extinction) Tommy grew up to know and like human beings. Unlike the black rhino, a tetchier type, the white or square-lipped rhino is almost as docile as a cow. I have often walked in among a group of two-tonne rhinos reclining on the grass, scratched their backs, sat on their armoured haunches and even slapped an injection into one of them. Tommy was so tame that he starred in a British Telecom television advertisement as 'Ryan O'Neal'. After I had confirmed that the young rhino was a perfect specimen, he was sold and went by sea to his new owners in Italy. I didn't know it at the time, but he was not destined for a zoo or safari park. He was joining a circus.

There are some animals which it is difficult to justify as in any way suitable for the life of a travelling circus. The rhino is one of them, but Tommy was at least in the best of circus hands. Circo Americano, one of the three finest circuses in Europe (the other two are Circus Krone of Germany and Circus Knie of Switzerland) take infinite care with the welfare of their animals. I had been called many times to attend to patients in the circus, particularly elephants of which they have an unusually large herd. My first work for Americano had been to remove a tumour the size of a water-melon from an elephant's upper leg. The operation had been a complete success, and I became accustomed to receiving phone calls from some city or small town in France, Germany or Italy where the circus was encamped, taking the next flight to the nearest airport, hiring a car and arriving to find everything prepared to the finest detail for examination and treatment of some sick animal. Afterwards, there was always the delight of seeing the show, the spectacular three-ring type unlike anything presented by British circuses, and then going with the Togni family, owners of the circus, to dine. Continental circuses know all the best eating-places on their touring routes and are generally old and valued clients of the *patrons*. If there are fresh white truffles or the first wild strawberries in town, they get them. All part of my life of veterinary gastronomy!

At Circo Americano, Tommy had happily acted as a living mobile platform for acrobats in the ring, though I never saw him perform. Then, on this day in June, with the circus come to town in Massa, he hopped it. For no apparent reason: curiosity, desire to stretch his legs or go in search of some fresh grass, perhaps. Tommy simply trotted out of the circus while he was being watered.

Two tonnes of good-natured, trotting pachyderm is as easy to stop as a Scorpion tank. You can't put the brakes on by grabbing its passing tail or standing in front of it, arm raised traffic-policeman style. A rhino is very short-sighted and doesn't even look at what it charges. Guided by acute senses of smell and hearing, it just puts down that horny head and goes.

With circus workers in full pursuit, Tommy went through Massa town centre, charging nobody, injuring no passers-by, simply a rhinoceros going AWOL, savouring no doubt the aromas of bread and garlic and chicory as he trotted past the food shops and ignoring the familiar human voices, barking dogs and honking motor cars. To the gawping citizens of Massa this was a fine *commedia*. Two policemen who had been standing, aimlessly smoking, in front of the parish church joined the band of circus men as they puffed by in hot pursuit. Action! In Massa! The honour of the *polizia*!

Gradually Tommy began to tire, and he slowed to a walk. Flavio Togni, in command of his staff, told them to hang back. He calculated that when Tommy had had enough, he would come to a halt. With familiar encouraging words, and by producing the apples that he'd stuffed into his pockets when he saw Tommy making off, the rhino could then be coaxed into the wagon that was already following slowly half a kilometre behind. The main thing was to avoid harassing or panicking the animal. Flavio had dealt with such escapers among eleph- ants in the past, and the 'softly, softly' patient approach had always been rewarded. He told the two policemen who insisted on leading the pursuers what he planned to do. 'Don't get in the way, don't do anything rash, don't "push" the beast. We know what we're doing and there's no danger to anyone if we just take it easy.' Another kilometre, and Flavio guessed Tommy would run out of steam.

It was at this point that the *carabiniere* (no lover of the civilian police whom, like most of his colleagues, he considered to be the Italian versions of Mr Plod) surveyed the scene from his cover in the vineyard. I can only imagine what he was thinking, for later his superiors would not let us talk to him about what subsequently happened. The monster was walking past him now, and it looked as if the two policemen were going to take a pot at it with their hand-guns. He could see how the local, nay the national papers, perhaps even the *Corriere*, and television too, would report it. Dangerous killer rhino wreaks havoc in Massa!

The *carabiniere* rose to his feet and emerged from the vine leaves. He clicked the safety catch of his nine-millimetre sub-machine-gun to 'off'. Flavio and the other spotted him immediately. 'It's okay, *signore*,' shouted the circus boss, 'every- thing's under control. We'll have him caught in a few minutes.' The rhino was now walking away from the *carabiniere* at an even slower pace.

'But the photographs, the interviews on television tomorrow will all be of that pair of flat-footed, parking-ticket *contadini*!' thought the *carabiniere* perhaps. 'Such a creature cannot be taken dead or alive by one of them. What will folk in Massa say when they know that I, Lorenzo, was there when the monster rampaged through the countryside, and did not act?' The *carabiniere*'s sense of duty to the good people of Massa had never blazed so fiercely. He lifted his gun and, pulling the trigger, sprayed the rhino with bullets. It was the first time he had fired the weapon in anger and he felt like the good-looking guy in 'Miami Vice'.

Tommy shuddered briefly, stopped walking but didn't fall. When Flavio came running up to him he even accepted an apple. Thin trickles of blood ran down from a number of small holes in his dusty grey skin.

La commedia è finita.

Accustomed as I am to off-beat opening lines when I answer the telephone – 'The dolphin's swallowed a football' or 'I think there's a vampire bat in the loft of my house in Bagshot' – Flavio Togni's 'Doctor, our rhino's been machine-gunned' took my breath away. He quickly told me about the shooting. 'We need you to come and get the bullets out of him – or he'll die!'

'Load him with penicillin and pick me up at Pisa airport,' I replied.

Apart from a few animals that had been peppered with shotgun pellets, I had no experience of gunshot wounds in exotic animals. As I packed some rhino anaesthetic, surgical instruments and emergency drugs into The Bag, I reflected gloomily on the impossible task ahead. No chance of X-raying to pinpoint the position of the bullets – even in the large animal clinic of a modern veterinary teaching hospital, the X-ray machines couldn't penetrate such massive creatures. And I knew how frustrating it was to try to track foreign bodies blind through their entrance hole. The natural movement of the muscles quickly and often progressively changes the position of an object such as a sliver of glass or metal. Searching for broken hypodermic needles in the old days, before they were laminated, could take hours in a small animal even if you started at once right at the spot where the needle went in.

But bullets – the plural was appropriate in Tommy's case – could travel no one knew how deep in rhino tissue, and they didn't necessarily travel in a straight line. Flavio had said they were nine-millimetre low-velocity bullets; perhaps they were lying just beneath the skin. If they were, was it really necessary to go after them? So many questions, so few answers.

*

My pessimism deepened as I sat on the BA flight from Heathrow, surrounded by summer holiday-makers. 'Have you been to see the Leaning Tower before?' asked the jolly lady sitting next to me, slugging back one Bloody Mary after another.

'Progfog,' I replied. 'Progfog.'

'Er . . . Pisa . . . *Have you been to the Leaning Tower before?*' She enunciated the words slowly, clearly, loudly in case I was both an idiot and a foreigner.

'Progfog blatch. Progfog,' I repeated.

The jolly lady nodded sagely.

'Oh, I see *you don't speak English. Ingleeeeesi?*'

'Progfog.' If necessary I can keep this up for a long time.

Smiling sympathetically, the jolly lady returned to her Bloody Mary, and didn't say another word.

My imaginary language is a boon when travelling by air. It gives me peace when I need to think. Headphones serve the same purpose on longhaul flights. But the more I thought about Tommy, the more doubtful I felt. What a pity Dr Wolpickel didn't exist!

Two years earlier I'd been telephoned by a man who introduced himself as Mr Jones, a Baptist minister from South Wales. 'Hello, is that Dr Taylor?'

'Yes.'

'I wonder if you could help me. I'm trying to trace a colleague of yours, Ulrich Wolpickel.'

'Who?'

'Wolpickel. Ulrich. You *are* David Taylor, the zoo vet, aren't you?'

'Yes, but I'm afraid I don't know any Wolpickel.'

'He's a zoo vet. German. Specializes in brain operations on rhinoceroses.'

'*What?*'

The minister went on to explain. A year before he'd helped out a German tourist who claimed to have had his money and belongings stolen while on a cycling holiday through the valleys. He found him a bed for the night, a change of clothes and some cash. The German was a charming, cheerful character. He told Mr Jones how he was a veterinary surgeon and that his main line of work was surgery within the skull of the rhino, and that he had originally been inspired to go into the zoological field after reading my first autobiography, *Zoo Vet* which was published in German under the name *Ein Herz für Wild Tiere*. Wolpickel stayed with the minister and his wife for a week. They all got on famously. He went to the chapel with them, and reinforced the singing of the thin congregation with his loud and not unmelodious voice. The week stretched to a month. The minister and his wife found themselves growing very fond of the nice young German vet who did such fascinating work, and when he one day announced that he must return to Germany to attend to a particularly sick rhino, they provided him with a further £150 on top of the £800 he'd already borrowed from them, and looked forward to seeing him, as he promised, in a fortnight's time when he would be back in Britain to have a meeting with David Taylor on certain advances in rhino surgery, and to repay his debts to his good Welsh friends. As you will have guessed, that was the last they saw or heard of the amazing Dr Wolpickel. Of course, he'd left an address, but it turned out to be non-existent. And when they checked via Directory Inquiries, there was no one with the name of Wolpickel in the town of Soldau, which was where he claimed his family home to be.

A year went by and still the Reverend Mr Jones and his wife continued to believe that there must be some innocent explanation. Maybe Ulrich was snowed under with brain-damaged rhinos. Or he had had a nervous breakdown after too many long hours at the operating table. Eventually, recalling Wolpickel's frequent references to me, the minister looked me up in the local library and telephoned. It was surprisingly difficult to persuade him that he had been well and truly conned.

'But he talked so knowledgeably about exotic animals, particularly rhinos. About surgery. About the anatomy of their skulls.'

'How do you know he wasn't talking nonsense, Reverend?'

'It sounded so correct.'

'He's a fraud, plain and simple.'

'Then how did he come to know so much about you?'

'From the books – easy.'

'And you are *sure*, Dr Taylor, that there is no German vet working on rhinoceros brain surgery?'

'Mr Jones. Firstly the skull of the rhino is so enormous, thick and complicated that no one, anywhere, has ever performed brain surgery on one. Secondly, rhino brain diseases, ones that conceivably *might* require surgery, are very, very rare. I've never come across a case. If Wolpickel, or whatever he was really called, ever tried to make a living out of rhino brain surgery he'd go broke!'

'Well, like I said, he didn't have any money.'

The naive and Christian gentleman couldn't believe it and, when at last the conversation ended, I'm sure he went away still doubting my explanation. Yes, a real Dr Ulrich Wolpickel could have been just the man for Tommy, I mused as we touched down at Pisa airport.

The *Daily Mail* had got there first, and a reporter and photographer were waiting with a car. Flavio and his men were busy tending to Tommy. They'd got him back to the circus without any trouble and he was apparently on his feet, though a bit groggy.

'The police and the *carabinieri* are squabbling like cat and dog over who fired,' said the reporter as we drove flat out for Massa. 'They haven't yet worked out whether it's a matter of guilt or glory.'

There was absolutely nothing glorious about the scene that confronted me when we arrived at the circus. Tommy lay dead. He had collapsed twenty minutes earlier. My sadness was overwhelmed by anger at the tragic stupidity of the affair. It wasn't the first time that escaped zoo or circus animals had been needlessly slaughtered by over-zealous police or militia men.

Although I was convinced that there was little, if anything, that I could have done for Tommy, and a full post-mortem in the circus field was impossible, I decided to probe the gunshot wounds to see whether I could locate any of the bullets. There was one wound behind the right ear, another that penetrated the ear flap and four scattered over the right thigh. In addition there were the marks of three ricochets. The most lethally placed bullet was the one behind the ear. Cutting with a scalpel, I searched for it. I followed its track as deep as I could, but didn't find it. It had most likely lodged somewhere at the base of the skull. The other bullets had also travelled so deep and so tortuously that I had no better luck in finding any of them. There was nothing more to be said or done. Disconsolately I flew home.

Later in that year, I laid my hands for the first time on the rarest and most enchanting of rhinos under quite different circumstances. Millionaire, gambler, eccentric, John Aspinall is regarded by many zoo men as a maverick. Maverick he may be, but a brilliant one, and he has established at Bekes-bourne, near Canterbury and Port Lympne, overlooking the Romney Marshes, two of the most important zoological collections in Europe. His breeding group of gorillas is arguably the best in the world and yields enough offspring each year for the planned reintroduction of complete family groups into the wild to be practicable in the not-too-distant future. Off public view there are facilities where endangered wild cat species can reproduce in tranquillity, and his elephant herd will also begin expanding naturally, for unlike many zoos who are unable or unwilling to keep elephant bulls, potentially the most dangerous of mammals, Aspinall has spent the time and money on building the necessary installations for the proper handling of such giants. He's often been attacked by the media over the series of accidents, some fatal, at his zoos. But in almost all the incidents there has been little scientific justification for the criticisms which have contained more than a little of the bile of envy and *schadenfreude*. Aspinall, friend of

Lord Lucan and host to the mega-rich at his Curzon Club, is just too damn clever by half, but for me he's a uniquely effective zoo owner. Only his frequent Sunday-afternoon frolicking with his full-grown tigers and gorillas in front of the public do I regard as foolhardy. Apart from the risk, small though it may be with animals who have regarded him as their dominant leader since they were babies, it is a bad example to the visitors. If 'Aspers' can get away with wrestling with a tiger, might it not be okay for some young buck to impress his girlfriend by vaulting the safety barrier and sticking a hand through the wire mesh to stroke a king of beasts?

In recent years, one of Aspinall's most significant projects has been the rescue of the Sumatran rhino. As well as the better-known rhino species in Africa and India, there are rarer and even more threatened forms which have their homelands in south-east Asia. They are the Javan and Sumatran rhinos. There are only about fifty of the former and a hundred or two of the latter left in the world.

With the blessing of the Indonesian and British governments, Aspinall has ploughed millions of dollars into the laborious and time-consuming process of capturing eight of the few remaining Sumatran rhinos, with the aim of setting up captive-breeding programmes in Djakarta and Port Lympne, with four rhinos being sent to each place. After almost two years and many expeditions by his staff in the Indonesian rain forest, the first two animals were caught and brought to Kent. Chris Furley, who had been our assistant for six years in the Middle East and was still associated with our practice, was now Veterinary Officer for Aspinall's two zoos. When the Director of Howletts and Port Lympne (an excellent zoo vet in his own right who had qualified at Glasgow shortly after me) had to go to Africa on sick gorilla business, he asked us, as he often does in such circumstances, to take care of the health of the Aspinall animals while Chris was away. So when one of the Sumatran rhinos developed a bloated stomach, John Lewis, another of my assistants who had also done his

stint in the Middle East, went down with me to see what we
could do with these little-understood creatures.

I like all rhinos, but I fell in love at once with these
Sumatrans with their fuzzy, reddish hair and twin horns.

One impressive thing about the Aspinall zoos is the incredibly high quality and broad range of the animal food. The
best of Covent Garden, Billingsgate and Smithfield produce
ends up there. The chimpanzees and gorillas eat prime condition exotic fruits, some of which I cannot name. The elephants and rhinos, the tapirs and the hunting dogs, are the
gastronomes of the zoological world. Every Monday is particularly special; then John Aspinall leads a small group compris-
ing his Director, Curators and Veterinary Officer round the
two zoos. It takes all day and is a sort of royal progress. He
inspects, discusses and expands upon each animal and – and
this is his delight – he hands out titbits, eagerly anticipated,
to every one, personally. Specially baked fresh bread and
chocolate bars for the rhinos and elephants. Choice meat for
the hunting dogs. Rare fruits and vegetables for the apes.
When he ran the Curzon Club, it was, and I suppose still is,
the rule that the high rollers at the tables were provided with
a lavish array of refreshments throughout the night. Whatever
they might fancy, their most outlandish potential whim, would
be catered for. A pricked pomegranate in Krug Imperial
for Kashoggi? Iced persimmons, quinces and guavas for the
Sultan of Brunei? Onassis feels like four ounces of Beluga
caviare on green limes and woodcock eggs at 3 a.m? At once,
sir, with our compliments. So every night the Club, like its
major competitors in the world of bored greed, had to be
provisioned with the finest fare, just in case His Majesty, His
Highness, or His Bankroll might feel like it. Consequently,
the following morning, there was a mountain of delectable
goodies that had not been summoned by the fickle palates of
the Great and the Not-So-Good. John Aspinall had all of it
sent straight down to his zoos. The casinos not only made the
money that funded his real love, the animal collections, but
did chimpanzee take-aways as well. I wager there are gorillas

in Kent who would make wonderful inspectors for Egon Ronay and could debate for hours the relative merits of Chilean or Israeli cherries.

John Lewis and I had the opportunity to see this cornucopia in action while we were treating the Sumatran rhino and trying, to put it bluntly, to make the animal fart its intestinal gas away. My lasting memory is of the way in which these creatures would take a whole sweet melon in their mouths and by sheer jaw pressure crush it. Juice exploded out of their lips in a golden shower that jetted in all directions and the ripe pulp was swallowed with audible murmurs of pleasure. Another one, please! The rhinos took melons as you would eat grapes. Watching the Sumatran rhinos I couldn't avoid thinking of Tommy. For sure, these animals wouldn't end up as acrobatic springboards riddled with bullets.

3 White and Wonderful

In Africa, the albino buffalo shares the sanctity of the elephant.
Sir Edward Burnett Tylor, *Essays on the History of Man*

'I am black, but comely, oh ye daughters of Jerusalem' goes a line in the Bible's Song of Solomon. Biologically speaking, black or dark brown pigment, in the form of melanin, is very useful stuff and to be born without any of it at all can be, for certain individuals, a black day – if you will pardon the expression.

Albinism – total lack of pigmentation – occurs, though very rarely, throughout the animal kingdom, including humans of all races. One in twenty thousand people is said to carry the recessive genetic factors that predispose to the condition characterized by white skin and hair, photophobia and susceptibility to ultra-violet-induced skin cancers. White foxes, blackbirds, opossums, monkeys, leopards, racoons, water buffalo and individuals of many other species have been recorded, and everyone is familiar with the albino breeds of domestic rabbit and mouse. Not being coloured like your fellows means, of course, that you stand out and lack the protection of natural camouflage; and the absence of colour pigment in the eye, exposing the blood vessels which give the characteristic red effect, make the delicate structures within that organ susceptible to damage by bright light.

My exotic patients have included a number of albinos over the years. There was Carolina Snowball, a striking pure-white bottlenosed dolphin caught off the coast of Carolina, USA. The other conventionally pale-grey dolphins with which she lived for many years in the Marineland treated her like any normal member of the group. One wouldn't expect any colour-bar among such highly intelligent mammals.

I have tended several albino king cobras – their deathly pallor made this most aggressive and dangerous of snakes seem even more forbidding – and on the children's television show 'No 73', where I presented natural history items for six years, I once met a charming albino toad, of the common or greenhouse kind, which had been found in Yorkshire. Although toads are shunned by most predators because of their ability to secrete a noxious liquid from their skin glands, they are preyed upon by some animals, and shining like a new golf ball among the petunias doesn't help such a small creature to maintain a low profile.

But the stars among my encounters with unusual white beasts were much bigger individuals. The first was, and still is, unique. Weighing around 180 kilos, most of it solid muscle, sweet or ugly-faced according to your taste, and the unofficial mascot of the City of Barcelona, he goes by the Spanish name of Copito de Nieve – Snowflake. Fragile, light and melting – he is anything *but*! Snowflake is a macho male gorilla. Not as white as an albino mouse, his shade is rather a pale apricot, particularly on hairless parts like the face, where the blood vessels glow through the skin.

Gorillas can live to about thirty-five years in the wild, and fifty years in a zoo. Snowflake was probably born around 1962 and so when Barcelona Zoo contacted me in 1986 he was a middle-aged gentleman. His parents were normally pigmented gorillas, but by some freak juggling of Snowflake's genes at the moment of his conception, he was destined to be different. His tragic early life was an all too typical one. Poachers in Guinea killed his parents in order to eat the meat, sell their heads and feet as tourist curios, and put up the baby for sale to a zoo or even as a pet. His unusual lack of colour made him even more of a prize; like thousands of little, frightened, pining orphans which have followed him down the same Via Dolorosa, he was sent to Spain where customs control of exotic imports was, and to some extent still is, remarkably lax. He was two or three years old when this latterday parody of the slave trade in those other Africans was played out and he arrived in a box, almost dead from malnutrition and neglect, at the zoo in Barcelona. Don't think that such traffic has yet been totally abolished. Dr Luera, the zoo's veterinarian, skilfully reared the little gorilla in his own home and Snowflake grew into a celebrity among zoo animals, the only albino gorilla that had ever been seen.

As a mature adult (one could hardly call him a silverback, the usual term for fully grown normally pigmented male gorillas because of their cloak of silver-grey hairs) he was in every respect other than skin tint a thoroughly normal gorilla – totally vegetarian, with that enigmatic, brooding character, less mercurial and frenetic than the chimpanzee and without the tranquil oriental philosophy of the orang-outang. He became in due course lord of the Barcelona gorilla family and fathered twenty-one healthy baby gorillas – but all of them in standard issue, run of the mill, black. Which was only to be expected. Shuffling the genetic codes in a fertilized gorilla egg throws up an albino rather less often than the bank is broken in Monte Carlo.

But with Snowflake due to approach the autumn of his life, it couldn't be assumed – still fertile though he was – that he would go on reproducing, like Charlie Chaplin, into his dotage. Barcelona Zoo were determined to preserve the possibility of producing another albino gorilla for as long as possible. I supposed they hoped to recreate the great blaze of publicity that had attended Snowflake's arrival.

Some animals that are freaks of nature, wild-born or contrived by humans, continue to be greatly prized. Though their peculiarity confers no fundamental scientific value, many people, including some zoo directors, possess a touch of the old carnival sideshow mentality. White gorillas, lion-tiger hybrids, dolphin-whale crosses and two-headed snakes, are all potential crowd-pullers, but don't *mean* any more than the bearded lady of times gone by. Gorillas are marvellous beasts under grave threat of extinction, but I don't find a gorilla made any more marvellous just because it lacks normal pigmentation. Barcelona Zoo had come up with the idea of a sperm bank, preserving Snowflake's semen and its contained genetic blueprint for years after his eventual demise in deep freeze. By diluting the stored semen and using it in carefully controlled amounts through artificial insemination, Snowflake might go on posthumously trying to throw Snowflake Junior well into the next century. To that end, they wanted me to extract a quantity of semen from him which would then be treated by a medical institute that specialized in human test-tube baby work. It would be endowed with a kind of chill immortality by being frozen at minus 79 degrees Celsius.

Artificial insemination, and the associated techniques of diluting and storing semen, were developed in animals long before being applied to human beings. Centuries ago, the Arabs collected semen from mares by inserting sponges into their vaginas. An Italian scientist anticipated today's deep-freezing of semen by experimenting on the effects of snow mixed with stallion semen in the eighteenth century. Artificial insemination and embryo transplantation are nowadays highly important and complex fields in animal reproduction, both agricultural and zoological. The techniques of semen collection vary from species to species. Giant condoms can be used on horses, and artificial vaginas are generally employed with bulls and water buffalo. Diluting the semen immensely increases the number of females that can be inseminated with it but it must be protected from the effects of the extremely low temperatures needed to preserve it for years; these necessitate all manner of chemical cocktails being added to the collected specimen, and each species has its own particular requirements. Among the diluents that can be used with semen are such things as coconut milk, tomato juice, honey, egg yolk, milk and, particularly good at stopping the poor little spermatozoa from getting frostbite, glycerol.

To take the semen from Snowflake would require me to use electro-ejaculation. This entails inserting a probe into the rectum at just the right spot in relation to the prostate gland and the nerves which trigger the muscular contractions of ejaculation, and applying a brief pulse of electric current. Though not dangerous, it is unpleasant for the patient (or so I am assured by the man who custom-built our probes for various sizes of animals; he assiduously tried out the one made for great apes on himself – without, of course, any anaesthetic). Snowflake would have to be given a general anaesthetic – after all, even for the best of reasons, bull gorillas don't take kindly to zoo vets walking up and sticking something that looks rather like a black plastic truncheon into their fundament.

The Barcelona zoo veterinarians had little experience of, and considerable apprehension about, anaesthetizing the most valuable (after the giant pandas I take care of in Madrid) animal in Spain. The responsibility for the operation would be wholly mine.

Twenty years had passed since I 'knocked out' my first gorilla, one of the pair that had arrived at Belle Vue, Manchester, just before the fine new great ape house was opened by comedians Morecambe and Wise. Since then I'd not had any problems, idiosyncratic reactions or circulatory collapses in inducing controlled, temporary oblivion in these mighty primates. A flying dart filled with one of a range of special concentrated anaesthetic solutions and fired from a blowpipe or gas pistol would have the biggest gorilla sleeping like a baby within five to ten minutes. There was no reason for me to suppose that Snowflake would be any different from an ordinary gorilla under anaesthetic *but* . . .

I made arrangements to perform the electro-ejaculation on a morning in June, and asked Antonio-Luis García del Campo, my friend and colleague at the Madrid Zoo, to meet me in Barcelona. There's no veterinary surgeon in Spain that I trust more as a collaborator during surgery. Together we had operated many times on pandas, elephants, komodo dragons, tigers and much else. Quick, strong and resourceful, he's the man to have beside you when, for example, you're blood-sampling rare Mhorr gazelle at night in a garden in Almeria with the only source of light a flickering cigarette lighter, or when an even rarer okapi collapses under general anaesthetic and for long minutes won't respond to your antidotes. Antonio-Luis was, and is, my ideal Number One at times like that.

Although such operations on unusual beasts might sound more taxing than their equivalent on domestic animals, I recall many hundreds of surgical cases at the Milnrow Road surgery in Rochdale where the patients were cats and dogs and occasionally rabbits, which gave the young vet I then was as much worry, and demanded as much nervous energy, as anything we tackle nowadays on dolphins or gorillas. And if I fail now, I don't normally have the added strain of facing the distraught owner of Fido or Felix and bearing sad tidings.

I walked with Antonio-Luis through the pleasant old-fashioned city zoo set in a park close by the Barcelona waterfront. We stopped to look at the killer whale, plump and gleaming like a blow-up plastic replica of himself, and now fully recovered; the last time I'd seen him was when he was being bullied by a tyrannical male dolphin only one-tenth of his weight. Typically, the killer whale had constantly turned the other cheek when teased and bitten by the dolphin, even though one snap of his powerful jaws with their long conical teeth would have stopped his tormentor – permanently. When I examined the whale he was covered with shallow tooth-marks. Although none of them was by itself a serious wound that haemorrhaged profusely, the sum total of dozens of lacerations, each losing a little blood, had produced a profound anaemia. And the poor whale was sore and stiff into the bargain. It was the dolphin form of the Chinese 'death of a thousand cuts' and I was in no doubt that the meek forbearance of the whale would shortly end in its death if something wasn't done at once. I had the dolphin, protesting loudly with angry squeals and chirps, moved the same day and set about relieving his victim's symptoms with analgesics and anabolic hormones concealed within the daily ration of herring and mackerel. The set smile of the bottle-nose dolphins that we find so engaging can sometimes conceal a deadly purpose.

When we walked over to the great ape house we found it to be crammed full of people. The zoo was apparently going to make the electro-ejaculation of their star animal a major media event. It had been decided that instead of operating in the zoo's veterinary clinic, I should work in the covered visitors' area in front of the windows through which Snowflake and his family could normally be seen going about their daily business. Tall television light stands ringed the table draped in green cloth. This was an operating *theatre* indeed – with emergency transfusion drips, oxygen bottles, instrument trolleys, gas machines and suction apparatus as the props.

'*Estamos en un circo!*' gasped Antonio-Luis when he saw the tight press of journalists, photographers and cameramen encircling the floodlit table. And beyond the expectant audience of *Homo sapiens* in the front stalls, a line of female gorillas and their young were squatting, as it were in the dress circle, noses flattened to the armour-plated windows and mesmerized by the feverish activity of these other apes. Snowflake, of course, was nowhere to be seen. He was in his sleeping quarters, unknowingly waiting for his anaesthetic dart.

Rendering him unconscious with the double-strength ketamine (we have a pharmacist in Yorkshire who specially concentrates this invaluable anaesthetic for us) went according to plan and he was then carried on a stretcher by six sweating keepers down the passageway and into the tumult. To make way for the mighty albino, lying like a dead caliph on his bier, two security guards with whistles and batons went ahead. Immediate uproar! Constellations of flashbulbs exploded, the crowd rocked and swayed as each individual pushed to get close to the sleeping giant, and the hot air, growing steadily hotter from the glare of the lights and the mass of human flesh, was filled with execrations, mainly in Catalan but with the occasional Castilian '*coño*', '*mierda*' and '*hijo de puta*' distinguishable. The noise was deafening and continuous.

Antonio-Luis and I, following behind the stretcher, found ourselves left behind for, though the crowd was forcibly parted to allow Snowflake's royal progress, it at once snapped shut when the two rear bearers went through.

'*Sacredenundondelaris!*' roared my companion, using the mock-Spanish exclamation that he loves and which I heard as a boy on a Dick Barton radio programme and taught him when we first met.

'*Por favor*, let us pass. *Por favor*, we are the *veterinarios!*' I shouted to the backs of a hundred heads. Snowflake was now lying *unattended* on the table. Suppose something happened – his tongue fell back and blocked the airway or his heart began to flutter!

'*Por* bloody *favor – soy el veterinario inglés. Permitenos pasar.*' To no avail. All eyes and ears were focused on the magnificent leading actor in the drama, lying there supine with his Falstaffian beer-belly and utterly tranquil apricot-coloured face.

As I have said, Antonio-Luis is an invaluable Number One. With the audience still between us and our patient, he decided to rely no more on exhortation. A basketball player of international class, he saw a chink between two pairs of shoulders in the back row of the crowd and smashed through, grabbing my arm in tow. Head down, I was dragged through the buffeting throng, almost losing my operating gown and having my shins kicked half a dozen times.

Roll of drums! Crash of cymbals! They would have been appropriate, for we emerged 'on stage' feeling more like knock-about clowns than veterinarians about to operate. But we were reunited with our patient. Ignoring now the cries of 'Doctor! *Please*, a photo by his head!' and 'Doctor, show us the thing you're going to stick up his bottom!', Antonio-Luis checked the gorilla's vital functions while I examined his genitalia. Everything my end seemed in order, and Antonio-Luis nodded to indicate that the pulse, respiration, capillary refill time and heart sounds were normal. I assembled the electro-ejaculator, plugged it in and selected the current strength. The journalists and paparazzi were by now at fever pitch and imbued with anatomical curiosity.

'I wanna get a picture of his *organ!*' screamed a woman reporter – one hesitates to imagine what sort of magazine she represented.

'Si, si, show us his *pistola*,' others shouted.

'*Donde está su polla?*' boomed a loud and vulgar voice. 'Where is his willie?'

Stone-faced, we bent over Snowflake's torso. Both Antonio-Luis and I knew that they were all labouring under a common misapprehension. How shall I put it? Gorillas are big and beefy, but their sexual organs are, by comparison, remarkably tiny. The really interesting biological question is why the genitalia of us, the naked apes, should be comparatively so large. With all set, I inserted the lubricated probe into Snowflake's rectum while Antonio-Luis held a sterile glass tube to the end of the animal's penis. Our actions induced sudden silence in the audience. While cameras continued to click furiously, their operators were struck dumb. The climax – in more ways than one I hoped – of our performance was at hand. I pressed the button to deliver a pulse of electricity. At once the lower muscles of the gorilla spasmed and his pelvis arched briefly. '*Ole!*' A man's voice broke the silence. But not a drop of semen flowed from his penis.

I adjusted the position of the probe and again pressed the button. Spasm. Erection. The penis was a blunt pink shrimp. But no semen. Six times I tried. Antonio-Luis even massaged the penis. And then on the seventh pulse – eureka! A globule of semen exuded from the minute organ, trickled down the tube – and promptly dried to a useless film in the heat of the arc-lamps! Never before had I needed to give so many pulses to obtain so small a sample.

Although he was unconscious of all this embarrassing pantomime, I decided that we had done enough to Snowflake. I was unwilling to prolong the anaesthetic and, after all, if a bottle is empty, it's empty. I withdrew the probe and said '*Finito!*' Snowflake could return to the privacy of his dormitory to sleep off the drug for an hour or so. Hubbub once more! 'Why? Why? Por qué? Por qué?' shrilled the reporters, 'What has gone wrong?' 'Is he impotent? Is he finished?' There would have to be a press conference as soon as we had washed.

Standing in front of the crowd of reporters now drawn up in a semi-circle, I explained what we had done and what the outcome was. For whatever reason, Snowflake was, as the Americans might say, 'clean out' of semen on that occasion.

'So what you are saying, Doctor, is that Snowflake was sexually active with his wife last night, ho ho ho!' crowed one journalist, scribbling this vigorously.

'*Si, es verdad!*' shouted the rest. It sounded to them like a suitably sensational explanation. I *wasn't* saying that, but they had stopped listening. Next day the papers were full of it, with some going so far as to depict me as a sort of mad English scientist doing unspeakable experiments with perverse sexual overtones.

'Don't worry,' said Antonio-Luis later, as we sat munching spider-crab with cold Monopole wine on the Ramblas. 'You know the Catalans – they had to have a foreigner to blame if Snowflake didn't satisfy their honour. It's just bad luck.'

'Next time, though, I think I'll arrange to have Snowflake kept away from his wives for a week or two before doing it,' I replied. 'It might improve our luck.'

White cats, not of the long-haired Persian kind, are a different matter. True albino lions *were* born in the Kruger National Park, South Africa, in 1960, but every year or two some little zoo or other excitedly publishes the news that its lions have had a litter of rare white lion cubs. Enter the television crews and journalists, all quick to believe, as indeed the owners do themselves, that this is something akin to growing a blue tulip or opening an oyster that hides a golden pearl the size of a squash-ball. And for sure the lions do have fur of creamy-white rather than the normal clay colour. For such white lions, seen in the heraldic devices of several noble houses, including the Dukes of Norfolk, a value of thousands of dollars each is put about. But all is not as it seems. Wait a few weeks, and the early pale shade darkens naturally and, long before they are three months old, the cubs are indistinguishable from other youngsters of less-celebrated birth.

White tigers, however, do exist. True albinos with pink eyes and no stripes have been recorded on at least one occasion, but beautiful so-called 'white tigers' of another kind are at present all the rage. White with blue eyes and dark stripes, they quite patently have too much pigmentation to be called albinos, and they are in fact an unusual chinchilla mutation. White tigers have been found in many parts of India, but it is those from Rewa with a creamy background to their coat which are the most famous. The Maharaja of Rewa began captive breeding of them in the early 1950s, and the first specimens to be seen in the West arrived at Bristol and Washington Zoos about ten years later.

In the past few years they have become star attractions in zoos and circuses in the USA and Europe, and can cost around $65,000 each, a hundred times more than an ordinary tiger.

Stukenbrock Safari Park, near Bielefeld in West Germany, has been a prolific source of interesting cases since I first became a consultant there in 1974. It was at Stukenbrock that Dr Ferdi Wurms and I washed the blood of a chronically sick elephant by passing it through an ozonizing machine. There, too, I had first seen a mysterious and still unexplained brain disease of big cats and, most dramatically, once come face to face with a tiger in a fog-swathed reserve that was thought to be empty of animals. There had been the exciting six-monthly hoof-trimming sessions in the main reserve with Fritz Wurms driving a Beetle at break-neck speed in zig-zagging pursuit of zebra and antelope while I fired tranquillizing darts out of the vehicle's window, and the fitting of plastic 'buffers' on to the sword-like horn tips of incorrigibly aggressive oryx that effectively stopped them from inflicting mortal wounds on other animals.

In 1987 Stukenbrock acquired a fine pair of one-and-a-half-year-old white tigers from Cincinnati in the United States. To house them a spectacular golden-domed Indian temple was built, surrounded by water, and containing excellent heated night quarters – and deep-freezes for a specially prepared brand of meat which was being imported from the United States. Joan Collins, the actress, performed the official opening of the cat house, and I was asked to go and check over the

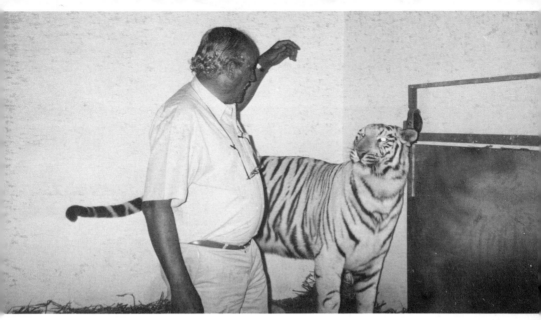

This white tigress isn't tranquillized . . . just friendly!

Measuring the blood-pressure of a sick lioness at Windsor Safari Park. (*White & Reed*)

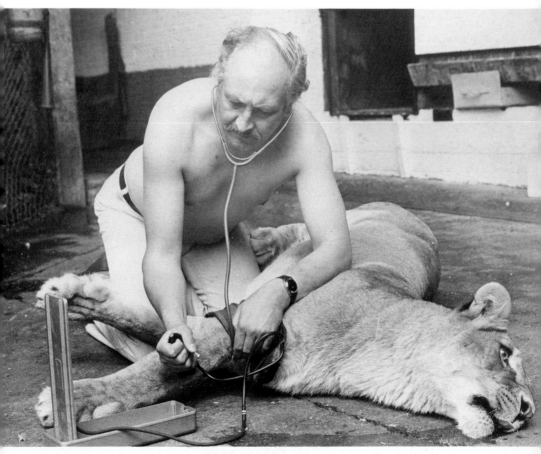

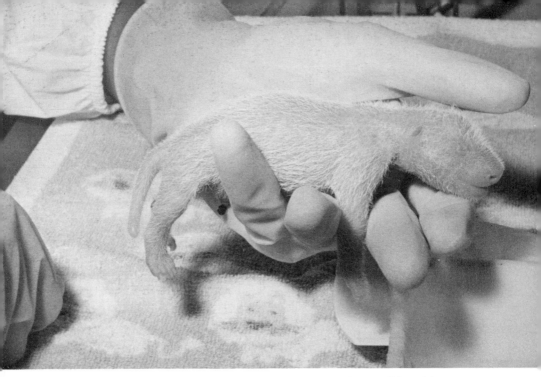

'Chu-Lin' when newly born: baby pandas began life without any black markings. (*J M. Martos*)

Taking unusual liberties. Giant pandas are not generally as cuddly and amenable as 'Chu-Lin', seen here at the age of one.

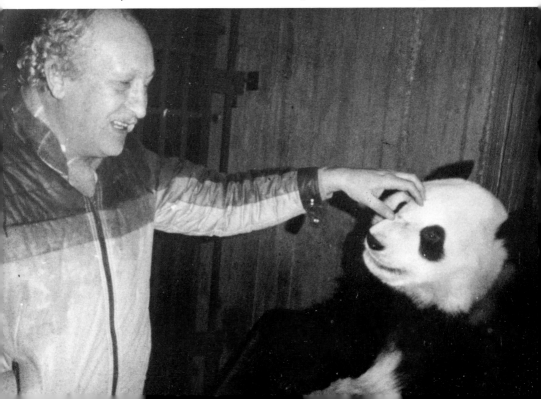

new arrivals. The pair of tigers were magnificent animals, adolescents who still retained some cubbishness, and as friendly and stroke-happy as any inglenook moggy. I've always had a rapport with tigers – possibly because I'm a cat person. Half the human race is cat-orientated and the other half dog-orientated, I believe. And cats, large or small, know which sort you are! But with tigers the interaction is enhanced by real communication. Say 'p-rr-rooch' to a tiger, and he'll answer you back. Try it next time you visit a zoo. 'P-rr-rooch-p-rr-rooch,' you go; 'p-rr-rooch-p-rr-rooch,' comes the reply. I am at once *in* with tigers. So it was with the white tigers at Stukenbrock. 'P-rr-rooch-p-rr-rooch,' then the reply and Fritz opened the door that led me into their sleeping quarters. Just like any of my old house cats – Lenin, Lupin, Tom, Buck-tooth and the rest – Savari, the male, and Saheba, his mate, came up to me and rubbed against my leg – the thigh, not the ankle in their case, nuzzled me with whiskery muzzles and uttered that other tigerish sign of friendship, a soft, gently plaintive 'wow'. Not that they were importuning me to open a tin of tiger-sized 'Kit-e-Kat' – just because they were *nice people*. And I am no animal sentimentalist – sentiment yes, sentimentality, no thank you. The animals were so fussy, so keen to play, that I had to do most of my examination on the move, walking slowly beside them with my stethoscope on their chests as they fawned and fondled.

They were in great shape except . . . Savari was breathing more rapidly, though no more deeply, than I expected. Twenty times a minute rather than ten. But the stethoscope revealed no unusual noises of the lungs or heart. Taking the temperature by popping a thermometer up the backside would not have been tolerated, even by these most affable of big cats.

'Both eating well?' I asked Fritz.

'*Jawohl*. Perfectly,' he replied, 'though I must say the stools are a little looser than those of the other tigers.' Stukenbrock has a fine collection of Bengal tigers and the curator, Herr Wilding, has a lifetime's experience of observing and caring for these most superior of wild felines.

With the heart and lung sounds apparently normal, I could find nothing to explain the raised respiration rate.

'Right. Tomorrow we'll do an X-ray of the chest and an electro-cardiogram,' I said, 'under light anaesthetic.' You can't do those examinations on fidgety, fussing tigers. There had been rumours emanating from the United States that white tigers were sometimes unpredictable when given anaesthetics. I couldn't find any firm information as to whether it was true, nor could I think of any physiological reason why that might theoretically happen. However, the majority of albinos cannot synthesize an enzyme called tyrosinase, which conceivably could alter the way the body handled injectable anaesthetics. I recall raising the matter of biochemical anomalies linked with albinism during a lecture by Dr Mulligan in my second year at Glasgow University. He didn't enlighten me, but said rather acidly, 'Bhoy, you're either a fool or a genius' – a quotation that was remembered and printed in the final year dinner souvenir book. And that was that. Anyway, as I've already said, white tigers *aren't* albinos. Surely they would be easy to knock out with one of my regular efficient drugs like ketamine or tiletamine. I would have the ECG and the radiographs done within fifteen minutes.

Taking a stool sample for bacteriological and parasite testing, I made arrangements for the tigers to be given no more solid food until after the anaesthesia and then went to spend the night at Hannelore's brother's house, just down the road in Sennestadt.

Next morning I was at the Safari Park by eight o'clock. A local equine veterinarian, who had agreed to bring a portable horse X-ray machine for the tiger examination, was already there with his assistant. The battery-operated electro-cardiogram was part of my travelling diagnostic gear. I set it up and calibrated it, checking that the roll of narrow graph paper was running correctly. With all prepared, a lungful of air puffed through a blowpipe sent a lightweight flying syringe with its content of ketamine into Savari's ham muscle. He didn't seem to notice the prick of the fine needle. Four minutes and twenty-two seconds later – I always time the injection period – the white tiger was fast asleep. I gave an injection of atropine to control drooling and protect the heart, and three of us then carried him out into the corridor of the temple where the equipment was waiting. Gently we laid the tiger down on his side on a large table. After putting on lead aprons and gloves we began taking a series of six X-ray films, adjusting the tiger's somnolent torso between each exposure in order to irradiate the lungs and heart from different angles. The exposed films were at once sent by car to be developed at my veterinary colleague's surgery. Throughout I checked the tiger's breathing, pulse and colour at regular intervals. Nothing was amiss. The respiration rate now was down to nine per minute and the heart was beating at a steady forty.

Next came the ECG. I connected four crocodile-clip electrodes, one to each of the tiger's limbs, and fixed them in place with adhesive tape. Leads from the electrodes ran to a plug, which in turn was inserted into the electro-cardiograph. I switched on. Immediately the hot stylus of the instrument began to inscribe a black line with a series of intermittent peaks and troughs on the graph paper that was steadily spewed out. The squiggly pattern represented the electrical activity in various phases of the white tiger's heartbeat. A valley too deep, a peak too rounded or an unexpected hillock in this innocent-looking cartoon of a range of mountains can signify a damaged valve, an enlarged chamber or one of the dozen other possible faults that can afflict the amazing non-stop muscle that is the heart. But the outline of Savari's ever-lengthening tracing formed that of a familiar horizon – a normal tiger heart with no nasty surprises.

I checked the breathing again with my stethoscope. One, two, three . . . the chest stopped moving. I looked at the ECG, still humming away. The stylus continued to write the same pattern. Pulse – good, strong. Breathe! There it was. Another breath, but weaker. The clusters of peaks on the graph paper began to group closer – the heart rate was accelerating. Shallow breathing now, irregular. One, two . . . three, four

. . . five . . . I touched the tiger's eyelids gently – no reflex blink. I tickled the ear – no reflex twitch. *My* pulse rate quickened. This was odd; by now the single dose of ketamine should have been wearing off and the animal beginning to curl its tongue, stir a leg, growl even. A full syringe of doxapram, to give a kick in the pants to the breathing centre in the brain, is always by my side when working with general anaesthetics. I slipped a dose into the foreleg vein and then pulled the tiger's tongue. It lolled out of the mouth.

'Is something wrong?' whispered Fritz. The Director, a tough and experienced animal man, was looking apprehensive.

'For some unexplained reason the breathing is sinking,' I replied. Just then the doxapram arrived at the brain and the tiger gave a deep breath. One, two . . . three . . . It was failing again. The ECG chart was now depicting a speeding heart, still functioning efficiently but very much aware of the reduction in oxygen quantity and trying to help as well as it might. More drugs by injection to boost the circulation. More breathing stimulators. Anxiously I watched the ECG with one eye on my watch and the hand under the tiger's groin taking his femoral pulse. One, two . . . fading.

'Oxygen from the maintenance shed!' I said. Fritz knew what I meant. Over his walkie-talkie he called up his head engineer. '*Schnell!* The cylinder of welding oxygen and a few metres of rubber tube.' A few minutes later a vehicle roared up and the oxygen cylinder was wheeled in. I put a towel over the tiger's head and led under it the rubber pipe from the cylinder. The gas hissed out as I turned on the valve. By now Savari should have been up on his feet, groggy, but more or less compos mentis. Yet he was as flat out as if I'd given a heavy dose of barbiturates, like in the old days. It's the liver that destroys the ketamine anaesthetic to clear it from the system. Suppose, I wondered, suppose that there *is* some idiosyncrasy, some biochemical quirk linked to the unusual colouring of white tigers, that makes them unable to destroy certain chemicals like ketamine. Cats aren't very good at the best of times in getting rid of substances like aspirin – which is why it's so easy to poison them with it. The rumours about white tigers and anaesthetics could turn out to be true!

It was a long day. Sitting there beside the unconscious tiger, monitoring its vital signs, turning it over every twenty minutes to prevent congestion of the undermost lung, massaging it, injecting it, testing the eye, ear and limb reflexes.

Two o'clock – the tiger's ear flicked for the first time when I tickled it yet again. Saint Francis, *ora pro nobis*! Four o'clock – as I opened the mouth to reposition the tongue that was in danger of falling back, it closed rapidly by reflex and I got my fingers out in the nick of time. We were winning! At a quarter to six when I nipped hard between two hind toes, the leg flexed. Fritz Wurms, who had stayed with me all the time, recognized the encouraging signs. He used his walkie-talkie again to order bratwurst and Malteserkreuz schnapps to be brought. We'd forgotten we hadn't eaten all day.

By nightfall, Savari was conscious again and able to sit on his haunches and lap water. But he wasn't back to normal until a further two days had passed. Thank God, though, I hadn't lost my first white tiger. The breathing was still faster than normal but the X-rays were as clear as the ECG traces. Nothing wrong with chest or lungs, but the tiger's loose stools turned into definite diarrhoea. Four days later the laboratory results arrived – the stools contained an abundance of salmonella.

Salmonella, post-Edwina Currie, has become an *in* word. Reading the newspapers one might get the impression that this notorious microbe is a newly arrived alien from outer space that is currently rampaging through the supermarkets, cheese-makers and chicken farms and making nervous housewives wonder whether there is *anything* that they can safely give their family to eat. But salmonella has been around for aeons. Members of this family of germs cause typhoid in humans and some of them, while carried principally by one host species, can cause fever, 'food poisoning' and serious diarrhoeas in other hosts. Among my patients I have found salmonella on occasion attacking nearly any animal you can mention – from giant pandas to camels, from crocodiles to flamingos. Although treatable with certain antibiotics, salmonella can, in some cases, strike quickly and lethally. Of all exotic animals, the elephant seems to me to be the most sensitive to this germ. After eating some contaminated food – say a stale ham sandwich proffered by a member of the public – there is sometimes so rapid a course with this disease that there is no time to diagnose or give therapy. An elephant with salmonella may go off its food, run a temperature and then die, all within a day or so and without there being time for it to show diarrhoea. On the other hand, a rat or a deer fawn or a pelican can carry the same strain of the germ with few or no symptoms for months on end. Tigers come somewhere in between. With them salmonella doesn't usually kill quickly, but an untreated case may end fatally after a few days or weeks.

Fritz Wurms was astonished when he heard the news. 'Everything of the best has been done for these tigers,' he exclaimed. 'The house is newly built, the hygiene, as you can see, is second to none, there are no pests like mice or rats in the temple, and the food is the highest quality.' He took me to the refrigerator and opened it to show the neatly stacked plastic bags of American chopped meat. It certainly looked more delicious than the frozen mince or hamburger meat in my local supermarket. 'Doctor – we're spending a fortune importing this stuff. All the way from the USA. Specially selected, vitaminized, certified – I've got half a ton of it in here, and there's five tons on its way by sea in a refrigerated container. What more can I do to keep the cats in good shape? And now you say there's salmonella. Where can it have come from?'

'I assume the tigers were fully examined and vaccinated by the American zoo vets before they came?'

'Of course. I have all the health certificates.' I knew the people in Cincinnati; they were first-class professionals. If they said the tigers were okay when they left, they were okay.

I walked round the temple with its moat of clean water and grassy lawn. All was sparkling new, no sign of pests, just as Fritz had said. Over-flying birds might have 'bombed' the outdoor area with salmonella-carrying droppings, but that seemed an outside possibility.

'Let me look at the meat,' I said finally. 'We'll do bacterial cultures on some samples.' Out of its bag and thawed, the American meat looked even better – to the naked eye needing only some raw egg, chopped onion, condiments and a couple of salted anchovies to make a perfect steak tartare. But the naked eye can't see everything. I took swabs from six packs of meat and sent them off to the German state veterinary laboratory. Half a week later the results came in. All were positive for salmonella, and the government vets weren't happy. Fritz Wurms was at once on the telephone to the meat suppliers in America, demanding an explanation and refusing to accept the consignment still at sea. 'What do you think you're doing, sending salmonella-contaminated meat to Europe?' he stormed. 'The state veterinary authorities are furious that so much food, certified as fit for consumption, should have arrived on their territory!'

'But the meat is fine,' came the reply. 'Salmonella is *always* to be found in such products, don't you guys know that?'

'If that's the case, why don't you mention it with the rest of the glorious promotional bullshit on the outside of the plastic packs?' demanded Fritz, slamming down the phone.

The American meat was never fed again, and the white tigers henceforth dined on the same meat as the other humbler tigers in the park, meat which was consistently found to be free of the salmonella bacteria. A course of antibiotic in the food eliminated the bacteria from the animals and the male's breathing rate subsided to normal. Both white tigers have continued to thrive well at Stukenbrock and with any luck will produce their first litter of white cubs within the next couple of years.

Since 1987 more white tigers have arrived in Europe, but so far I haven't had to anaesthetize another one. If and when

I am faced with the need to do so again, it will be with some trepidation. White tigers, like white gorillas, are different. I wonder how I'd fare with that most elusive deep blue-coloured tiger seen once in broad daylight in Fukien, China in the 1920s. Better perhaps – blue is my lucky colour.

4 Dolphins in the Dumps

The Dolphin fish . . . is a lover of man.

Erasmus, *Colloquia*

Abdel Nasser felt like a Pharaoh. *Humdilallah*! God had indeed been good to him. Only great, even greater things, could come out of this. One moment he was a bell-hop, the bottom of the heap, running, always running, carrying, shouted for, shouted at, for a few Egyptian pounds a month, and then, suddenly, he was a *star*! From time to time American tourists would come to the pool-side to admire his work, ask him questions. He'd had his picture taken with a grand French lady – although she declined to shake his hand afterwards and he'd overheard her say to her husband as they walked away that he, Abdel Nasser, smelled badly of fish.

Billah! He was the most fortunate of young men. Once, taking baggage to a room in the hotel, he'd caught a glimpse of a television set and the American programme that was running on it. It was Hollywood and adventure and *him* with his two amazing, magical beasts. He didn't know it, but the film was a re-run of an old 'Flipper' episode. Abdel Nasser, the lad given the name of the revered first president of the country, who lived in a slum near the pyramids, and who would drink a glass of dirty water straight from the Nile for a dollar to impress the tourists, Abdel Nasser, thin, consumptive-looking and often hungry, was the master of the two clever grey fish that in Arabic are called *darfel* and in English, dolphins.

He would never forget the morning earlier in the year when the Manager of the Meridien Hotel *himself* had called him to his office. Going up to the plush suite he'd been terrified – if he were about to be sacked, surely someone in personnel would simply have rung the head porter. To be summoned by Monsieur Speck was quite another matter – had some

visitor accused him of rifling luggage or gross impertinence?
It didn't make sense – even if he charged naked through the
dining room on a camel, the bell-hop would have been swiftly
dealt with by Personnel. But then, as he stood before Monsieur
Speck with his scrawny knees knocking inside the uniform
which he was now certain he would never wear again, he
heard the astounding words.

'Abdel Nasser – you're going to have to take charge of the
dolphins from now on.'

When he went back downstairs, it was almost enough to
make the young Muslim ask his friend, the assistant bar
tender, for a stiff *arak*. He made do with mango juice.

'*Hanni wa afia!*' whispered the bar tender. Good health and
prosperity – it certainly looked as if it was going to come the
way of Abdel Nasser.

When the luxury Meridien Hotel, situated on the bank of the
Nile in the centre of Cairo, had arranged with Monsieur
Linehard, a Swiss who owned some performing dolphins, to
bring a couple of them and some sea lions to spend a season
in the swimming-pool, no one doubted that it would be a
money-making sensation. The show would provide a new
source of entertainment for the hotel's guests, and draw in
crowds from among the well-heeled sections of that old strum-
pet of a city. Monsieur Linehard had for long been an anomaly
in the world of dolphins – a man with dolphins and no pool
to keep them in. For years he had moved his patient creatures
from one borrowed or rented pool to another. Detested by zoos
and marinelands, with their constantly improving facilities for
the care and housing of marine mammals, he was an odd-ball,
Mr 'Rent-a-Dolphin' who – as international regulations to
control the catching and keeping of dolphins were introduced,
beginning with the principal source, the United States, in the
1970s – somehow managed to find other, less particular,
sources of animals. Once he shipped a large consignment of
dolphins from Taiwan; most were dead within days of their
landing in Germany. The notorious minute glass 'dolphin

pool' beneath the stage of the Moulin Rouge nightclub in Paris housed some of Linehard's dolphins for many years. Later he had shows in Belgium, Italy and Spain and when these closed down, sometimes under a cloud of acrimony, he and his dolphins would simply move on. In the mid-1980s the Common Market countries began to take more interest in cetacean species crossing their borders. Permits were now needed and the scope for Monsieur Linehard, or anyone else, to pop up with a portable plastic pool, a tent and dolphins on a piece of waste ground in the middle of Madrid or Manchester was severely curtailed. But there are other countries, and Egypt is one of them.

At first all went well at the Meridien. The Linehard show attracted much attention. It looked as if everyone concerned was on to a money-spinner. Abdel Nasser, the bell-boy going about his duties in the hotel, occasionally had the opportunity to watch from afar. He marvelled at the way the European trainer waved his hands and made the fish do all manner of things. The man moved his arm and the fish would leap high in the air. Sometimes they didn't leap, and it seemed logical to Abdel Nasser that the fish did not then receive their reward of pieces of much smaller fish. Usually, if he stood for more than a minute gazing through a window at this fascinating scene – he wasn't allowed to go down to the pool area, which was fenced off for the paying audience – he'd receive a poke in the ribs from an under-manager and be told to get on with his bell-hopping.

In spring 1988, the Meridien and Monsieur Linehard fell out over matters which the courts in France and Egypt may one day decide upon, and the eventual upshot was that the sea lions and the dolphins were left in the hotel with neither Monsieur Linehard or any of his employees around to take care of them. The sea lions ended up at Cairo Zoo, but the dolphins stayed where they were – lazing around in the swimming-pool designed for tourists, and with the shows called off.

The Meridien Hotel is itself a miniature metropolis within a teeming, sprawling city where it is not uncommon to see a dead man or a dead donkey lying in the gutter, where, through numberless narrow, dust-carpeted streets, patchworked of gloom and glitter and lined by the smoke-blackened niches of artisans, barbers' booths, spice shops and cool mosques, the life of the Nile delta courses in all its colours and voices, its rags and gold bangles, its hennaed hands and tattooed Coptic crosses, its aromas of coffee, bread, *halwa* and dung. Here, hurrying by or sitting in doorways, are *fellahin* from the country, Muslim and Coptic townsfolk, Nubians, bedouin, Syrians, Levantines, Turks, Persians – and tourists. The Meridien town within a town is an island in this wondrous, pungent broth of a place whose multitude of staff will cook the best cheeseburger or *shish taouk* in town, instantly provide a secretary if you feel like dictating your will and launder your dress shirt or *dish-dasha* in a trice. They can attend with perfect efficiency to every need and whim of the diplomat from Algiers, the businessman from Paris, the honeymooners from Poughkeepsie – what they can't attend to is two male Atlantic bottle-nosed dolphins 'squatting' in the swimming pool.

For the first time in its life, the hotel found itself with two guests it couldn't handle. Worse, they were costing money, making none *and* occupying the human guests' rightful pool with the furnace heat of summer not far off. It would take a few days to sort things out and find somewhere else for the dolphins to go; meanwhile the hotel would do the best it could. Before the animals arrived special filtration equipment had been installed to keep the water clean – the hotel engineer knew which buttons to press. There was still an *ersatz* fish kitchen behind the row of pool-side cabins and they could continue to buy fish from the market. What they badly needed was a dolphin-keeper – someone to take some sort of care of the animals. Egyptian dolphin-keepers are as thin on the ground as Egyptian astronauts, so a member of staff would have to learn the hard way. Abdel Nasser was sent for. While the erstwhile bell-hop went trance-like to claim his kingdom – standing for long minutes by the pool looking down at the two squawking 'fish' and exploring his little kitchen with its knives, buckets and refrigerator full of mackerel – Monsieur Speck set about off-loading the animals. With any luck, Abdel Nasser would be back in front hall in a couple of days. The financial and legal aspects of the Linehard/Meridien dispute could be settled all in good time, but he couldn't afford to have the star performers living in their 'dressing room' at his expense. He knew that they were worth a lot of money; they would serve as collateral in hand for any claim he might make against the Swiss fellow.

But it wasn't as easy as he had foreseen. Dolphins, he found, aren't like fairground goldfish – they need filtered salt water and marine fish food, and transporting them requires special methods and people who know what they are doing. The offers he had from persons in Egypt, willing – indeed anxious – to take the dolphins, were hopelessly unacceptable. Garden ponds and a freshwater boating lake. The days stretched to weeks, and the weeks to months. Desperate by June, and with Monsieur Linehard irritatingly from time to time slipping into the hotel and watching from a balcony to see that his dolphins still numbered two, appeared alive, and were therefore at least being fed at no cost to himself, Monsieur Speck got in contact with marinelands overseas who might be willing to board the animals. Among them were Windsor Safari Park and Marineland Côte d'Azur in Antibes, France.

Michael Riddell, the English director in Antibes, replied to the request from Cairo in the only way he could. Yes, he would, of course, give the dolphins a home, *but* he would have to have an import licence from the French government and a guarantee from the appropriate French and Egyptian government ministries that he would not be involved in any legal wranglings with Monsieur Linehard, of whose exploits over the years he was well aware. A perfect, empty hospital tank was waiting for the dolphins in Antibes, together with expert staff, superb back-up facilities and myself and Andrew as veterinary surgeons. Michael had no desire to appropriate the two dolphins – he had enough of his own anyway – but he was more than willing to look after them until the business arguments in Cairo were settled; but only if he got the import permit and guarantee of no hassle. It was the same for all the major marinelands in Europe, operating now under governmental regulations. Nothing happened. No permits and no guarantees were forthcoming.

Abdel Nasser, no longer in bell-hop uniform, but affecting the style of the European trainer he had seen, wearing trousers and an old tee-shirt, was living virtually night and day with his 'fish'. He had become the envy of the other bell-hops, the assistant bar tender and the scullery workers. Even that Olympian figure, the maître d'hotel, once came down to the pool to *ask questions politely*! When he went home, the neighbours hadn't at first believed his story of being appointed Hotel Animal Trainer but they opened their eyes wide and exclaimed '*Wallah!*' 'By God!' when he passed round the polaroid photograph a visitor had given him that showed him standing next to a glamorous American lady in shorts and proffering a fish to a jumping dolphin. And he felt, as the weeks passed by, that he was getting somewhere with the animals whose names were now 'Nemo' and 'Limo'. Hand-waving seemed indeed to be the key, and Abdel Nasser did little 'shows' for himself, and sometimes even for a small crowd of hotel guests. Everyone seemed delighted, so it must have been going well, and though Abdel Nasser's shows were free of charge, once or twice he had a dollar or pound slipped into his fishy palm after the performance. The paradise promised in the Koran seemed pale in comparison to those summer days on the Meridien pool deck with Nemo and Limo more beguiling to him than any *houris*. Apart from the engineer who occasionally came to look at the filter machinery, the young Egyptian was left to himself. No interference. No orders. No bawlings out. The Arab saying is true, he would think to himself, as he cut the fish each morning – '*Allah karim*'. God is merciful.

By late autumn Monsieur Speck was even more desperate. Still Nemo and Limo swam in the pool by the side of the Nile, and somehow the British press had got hold of the story. The *Sunday Times* in particular was on the warpath, lambasting Linehard and calling for international action to save 'the abandoned dolphins in the Cairo hotel'. Abdel Nasser was still at his post, cutting his fish, 'training' his animals and doing the very best he could to keep them happy. Understandably, he was oblivious to the cloudy green water in the pool and the flies in his fish kitchen. Abdel Nasser had lived all his life by the black and turbid Nile where fish lived happily – he'd fished them – and weren't flies just living dust? You didn't *notice* flies unless you went to the abattoir during Ramadan.

November came and with an impasse in the relations between the Hotel and Monsieur Linehard, and the dead hand of bureaucracy on everyone's shoulder, the *Sunday Times* paid towards the expenses of sending a Zoo Check representative to Cairo to see what condition the dolphins were in. The Zoo Check man, a fireman who had worked at Windsor Safari Park years before, telephoned me in a state of high excitement. 'The dolphins are in terrible shape,' he told me. 'Bad water. Ill. Skin disease. I think they've swallowed something, the bottom of the pool is littered with bottles and other rubbish. Can you help?

'Do you think you can get some blood?' I knew that he'd watched me do it many times at Windsor in the old days. I also knew Cairo Zoo's vet had no experience with cetaceans.

'I'll try,' he replied.

'Even one cc is better than nothing. Take it to a hospital or private laboratory. I'll give you a list of the basic analyses. Then ring me back with the results.'

Next day he telephoned. He'd got a little blood, after a lot of effort, and I congratulated him. His problem had been finding anywhere that could provide him with blood-collecting tubes. My problem was that the results which he gave me didn't make medical sense. They were grossly, impossibly, abnormal. The Zoo Check man was doing his best, but it was impossible to know what proportions of his report were imagination, hype or plain fact. The lab reports didn't help.

I suggested some provisional treatment if, as the blood results indicated, the dolphins were infected with everything from tonsillitis to tuberculosis, but I felt uneasy about the whole situation. It was a bad mix. Linehard dolphins in an Egyptian pool. Bizarre blood results that couldn't be trusted. Well-meaning amateurs taking responsibility for the care and treatment of some of the most complex mammals in the world. And, accustomed as I was to long-distance telephonic veterinary consultation, I felt myself to be right out on a limb with this case. Someone had to take a firm grip on a situation which could now conceivably end in tragedy. Linehard's arguments with the Meridien didn't come into it.

The very next day Michael Riddell phoned me from Antibes, and what he had to say put a completely new complexion on the Nemo and Limo story. 'The French government will let us bring them in at last. We'll give them a home for as long as they need till things are sorted out permanently. The French Embassy, and the British, are working on the Egyptians. At this rate, by the time the Linehard/Meridien game comes to checkmate the dolphins could be long dead. I'm sending John Kershaw down to Egypt today. You go when he has had a chance to report back.' There at last was the firm grip. John Kershaw, the head trainer at Marineland, is one of the most experienced English dolphin men. Remarkably strong, though not heavily built, a fine linguist, resourceful and intelligent, he is the brother of Nik Kershaw, the pop star. His 'feel' for dolphins and other marine mammals, as I knew from working with him in Britain, Spain and Iceland, as well as France, is unsurpassed. If John said the Cairo dolphins were in trouble, they were in trouble. I've never known him exaggerate or underestimate the condition of his animals. John rang twenty-four hours later, at exactly the time we had arranged.

'What's the position?' I asked.

'Shitsville!'

'Meaning exactly what?'

'Filthy pool water, filthy fish kitchen for the dolphins (not

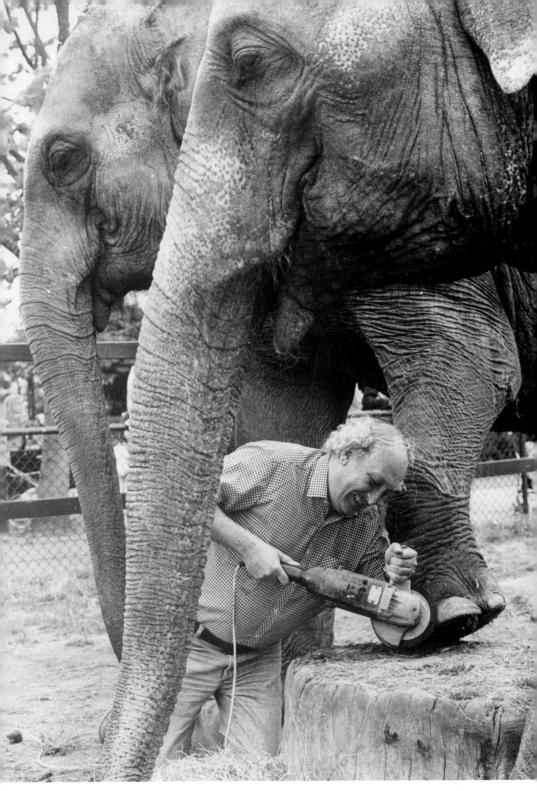

A zoo vet must be prepared to try his hand at chiropody! (*White & Reed*)

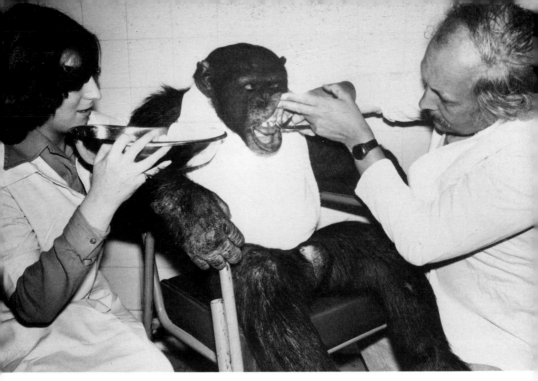

Suitably doped, an old male chimpanzee has a rotten tooth extracted. (*White & Reed*)

The rescue of the Cairo dolphins began after midnight, under conditions of great secrecy. (*Rex Features*)

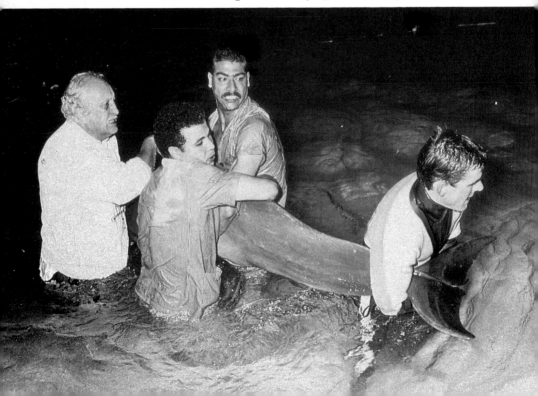

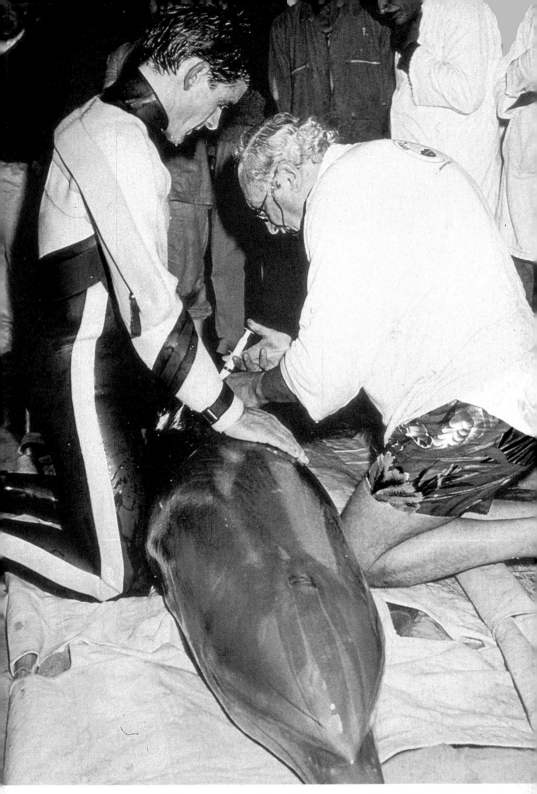

While John Kershaw steadies him, I prepare 'Nemo' for the flight out of Egypt. (*Rex Features*)

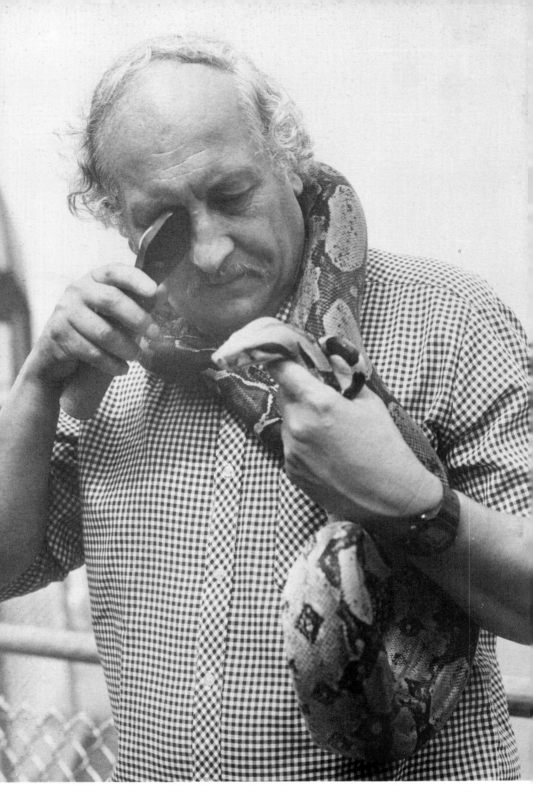

This snake at Chessington Zoo has some unsloughed skin still stuck to its eyeball. (*White & Reed*)

the hotel's – that's mega-luxury – and the kitchens are ace),
poor quality fish, dolphins in tatty condition, tails full of
pinholes where somebody's being trying to take blood, and
some poor, bloody Arab boy in charge of the whole *bordel*.'

'Damnation!'

'What should I do?'

'Take some more blood' (John can do this as easily as I
can) 'and get a proper blooming analysis – I'll be down in
two days. Meanwhile, try to change the water and get some
better fish – the hotel *must* have some for its restaurants.' I
needed the two days to go to Germany to examine a snow
leopard that seemed suddenly to be going blind.

On 17 November 1988 I flew to Cairo. The Meridien Hotel
employs a phenomenal 'fixer', Salem, who knows everybody
that matters, and he got me a visa, a place at the front of the
passport queue and through customs in a little under three
minutes. It was good to be back in the city, so rich in well-worn
character, down at heel, but bursting with warm humanity,
quite unlike the soulless kitsch of the Arab cities of the Gulf.
Within half an hour I was at the hotel, and being briefed by
John Kershaw over a pot of Turkish coffee.

He explained how the pool was now guarded round the
clock by burly security guards, that he had abandoned the
unsavoury makeshift fish kitchen used by the Linehard staff
and was preparing food for the dolphins at a sink and cutting
board set up in the open air, and, most important of all, that
Nemo and Limo were not in good condition, physical or
mental. 'When I first arrived they were utterly screwed-up
psychologically, with evil tempers. Bit me hard if they got the
chance. Behaved like a pair of lager louts!'

John had never encountered such bloody-minded dolphins.
We walked down to the pool and I was introduced to Abdel
Nasser, a lanky pleasant-mannered young man with close-
cropped hair, who looked to me none too healthy. It was dark
and impossible to inspect the animals, but the water was
visibly cloudy. 'It takes forever to change the water,' said the
dolphin trainer, 'and I'm sure the filtration isn't working

properly. When I dived I found the bottom of the pool littered with foreign bodies.'

'I'll do an examination first thing in the morning,' I replied. John's blood results from the local laboratory were as unlikely as the previous ones. I would take my own samples back to London.

'Any idea why the dolphins are so aggressive?' I asked. John waited until Abdel Nasser was out of earshot.

'It's him,' he said in a low voice. 'He was the cause. But you can't blame the bugger. He'd seen the Linehard's trainer apparently waving his arms and giving fish to the dolphins as rewards for well-executed behaviours. So when he took them over, Abdel Nasser imitated what he thought he'd seen. Waved his arm without any idea of the correct signals. Teased the animals by showing them fish and then denying it to them when, as happened ninety-five per cent of the time, they couldn't understand his body language. They didn't know where they were with him. He was the human with the fish, but he unwittingly tantalized and frustrated them. I watched him at it – innocent as the day is long. No wonder they became bolshie!'

So that was it. Dolphins quickly learn to associate a whole range of movements of the fingers, hand or arm with the request to perform particular 'tricks'. The fish pieces are given as a reward for a good effort, and a whistle if often used as a so-called 'bridging signal', blown at precisely the right moment to link the dolphin's actions with the prize, aurally. A dolphin hears things through the pinhole-sized ear orifices set behind the eyes and, more remarkably, through the tip of the chin and the armpits. The full sequence is signal, often very subtle, perhaps merely the movement of one finger (dolphins have good underwater and out of water vision), correct performance of the required behaviour by the animal, the whistle which in effect says 'well done that time' and, lastly, the piece of fish as a reward. Advanced training can omit one or more of these four phases, even including the giving of the reward. Dolphins love performing. Their biggest enemy, clearly evident in Cairo, is boredom.

'I'm doing all the feeding myself now,' John went on, 'not asking them to do anything, not trying to guess what Linehard's man's signals might have been. I'm just giving 'em lots of fish whenever they want it. And they're already beginning to calm down and recognize me as the friendly guy with a full bucket who doesn't give them any hang-ups!'

He had plundered the hotel's kitchens for their finest fish and Monsieur Speck, the Director, was more than willing to do anything that could stave off any more bad publicity about the dolphins, and that might possibly bring nearer the date of their departure. While we were at the Meridien, John and I lived like kings, on the house, and anything I needed for the animals was provided without demur.

The next morning was warm and bright; November is a great month to visit Cairo. There was a gentle breeze off the river and black kites were circling high in the sky as I went down to the pool, running the gauntlet of uncommunicative men in suits bulging with muscle and other objects who were on guard and had set up their headquarters in one of the cabins. The British press and a couple of television crews were already there. The pool was not very big, roughly circular with half of it about two metres deep and the rest half that. John had managed to get the water level dropped so that men could wade easily and help him catch my patients. Something the Meridien hadn't been able to find was a soft strong net, for us to use to sweep the animals into an area where John could seize hold of them one at a time. We had to make do with an old volleyball net. The Egyptian hotel workers who had been deputed to go into the water with John didn't seem to relish the task, and Abdel Nasser explained to me that they were not convinced that these 150-kilo torpedoes with curving dorsal fins weren't sharks. But they did what John instructed through an interpreter, and soon we had the two dolphins safely lying on an old mattress by the poolside.

I examined them from tip to tail, checked their chests with my stethoscope and took some blood from their tail-fluke veins. Nemo was thin, and had an area of pneumonia in the right lung. The cornea of his left eye was scarred by a healed ulcer and there were the typical scars on his flippers caused by using badly designed stretchers, or not positioning the animals correctly, during transport. Limo had similar flipper scars and an ulcer on the left eye. His weight was within normal limits. Both dolphins displayed the black dots denoting pox virus infection scattered over their skin. After the examination I gave Nemo some Ceporex for his pneumonia and then the animals were put back in the water. I looked round the 'dolphinarium'.

Over the low wall of the pool deck, I looked down at the bank of the Nile, the dark water swirling below me, washed-up flotsam drying in the sun and cats scavenging around the corpse of some small creature. The sink where John cleaned and cut his food was a vast improvement on the one that had formerly been used for the purpose but, as I watched, flies rose from the great river and homed in on the smell of the fish.

The dolphins had been there too long. The risks were too great, the conditions inadequate. And Nemo, if nothing else transpired, was suffering from pneumonia. I would fly back to London the next morning, courier the samples up to Oxenhope where Robert Turner, a pathologist and retired professor of human oncology, was now running our own small laboratory. Then I would make my decision.

My inclinations were, as I told Michael Riddell on the telephone, to move the dolphins to Antibes as soon as possible. Then we could give them the best of attention. Normally we would not consider transporting a dolphin that wasn't in perfect health; the Cairo animals seemed like the exception that proved the rule. If Michael could organize a fast aircraft across the Mediterranean, it would be just like flying a serious case of human accident or disease to a centre equipped to give the best treatment. Such mercy flights happen every day. Michael, who had once brought a healthy dolphin from Switzerland to Antibes in a private ambulance with police

escort, agreed. He would make the first moves in setting up
an air ambulance service for Nemo and Limo.

Back in England, Professor Turner's analyses confirmed
the fact that Nemo was indeed suffering from an infected lung
– for how long the pneumonia had been present was anybody's
guess. I rang Antibes to say that the transport must go ahead
without delay. Michael had by then arranged for Air France
to divert a Boeing bound for Marseilles from Djibouti via
Cairo in two days' time, and had already sent two padded
canvas slings for the dolphins down to Egypt by air. John, at
the Meridien, was busy organizing the construction of light
metal frameworks in which to suspend the slings as well as
fending off the increasing number of media folk who were by
now in full cry. Monsieur Speck and his executives were
arranging ground transport, minimum formalities and smooth
passage through the customs for the dolphins – we'd be leaving
during the night when it was cool for the animals and the
chaotic Cairo traffic was at its thinnest. Salem had the contacts. Palms were greased liberally. The hotel was also liaising
with the Egyptian government and French Embassy – we still
hadn't received official documents allowing the dolphins to
be exported to 'a place of safety' and there was a series of
meetings with lawyers handling the many legal aspects of the
affair. Monsieur Linehard's lawyers were also industriously
beavering away in the hope of blocking all our efforts to move
the animals.

By 22 November I was back in Egypt, prepared for a quick
turn-round. Arriving at 8 p.m., I hoped to be taking the
dolphins out of the pool about 2 a.m. the following morning,
at the airport with them by 3.30 a.m. and in Marseilles for
coffee and croissants at 9 a.m. Michael, typically, had arranged
for the Antibes fire brigade to send a vehicle to pick up the
dolphins at Marseilles and for six police outriders to slice
them through the traffic and down the autoroute to Marineland, blue lights flashing and sirens wailing. With any luck,
by 2 p.m. on 23 November, Nemo and Limo would be in their
new home relishing a few choice North Sea herring.

It was not to be quite like that. Worried faces greeted me at the Meridien, and I was hurried into a meeting with Speck and his lawyers. 'It's off,' the Director said simply. 'Linehard's lawyer has slapped an injunction on Air France. They cannot carry the dolphins.' This was serious. The legal battle might go on for months, if not years – what was to become of Nemo and Limo while the lawyers grew fat?

'Have you got the "place of safety" export permit from the government?' I asked.

'Yes, that came through. Though the opposition is going to protest about it in front of a judge tomorrow.'

That well-known ass, the law, seemed likely to kick poor Nemo and Limo in the teeth if things went on like this.

'So – if we could find some *other* airline to fly us out, they wouldn't be covered by the injunction?'

A lawyer nodded. '*If* you could find such a thing at this late hour.' Everyone agreed it was near impossible, but Monsieur Speck and his 'fixers' said they would try. Salem was sent for.

I went and ate supper with John. With both of us in a glum mood, the baked *garoupa* fish tasted of nothing. Then, suddenly, at ten o'clock, a waiter called me to the telephone. It was Monsieur Speck. Would we go to his office right away? He no longer sounded defeated.

'Great news!' he announced, as he shut the door behind us. 'We've got a plane! A 707. ZAS Airlines. A little outfit that runs mainly between here and Holland. We're in touch with their president. He thinks it's a great idea, will do it for free, and has ordered his staff to pull out all the stops. And what's more they'll go straight to Nice, not Marseilles!'

A miracle had happened. If this came to pass, we'd avoid the road journey from Marseilles to Nice. Marineland is only ten minutes' drive away from Nice airport.

'When do we go?' John asked.

'Our estimated time of departure is 4.30 a.m. Everything is arranged, *but* we must keep it top secret. If the Linehard lawyer gets wind of this, he'll drop an injunction on ZAS as well, even if it means waking some judge up in the middle of the night!'

The following half-hour was more like a gathering of SAS commandos planning a desperate mission. As soon as the last diner had left the restaurant, Speck would see that the lights were switched off, so that they did not illuminate the pool area through the windows overlooking it. The security guards would be stood down, the equipment ready for the Air France transport, including the lights which had been set up round the pool, would be taken away and stowed in an empty cabin, and all journalists and television crews (with the exception of one, which would be pledged to secrecy) would be told that, because of the injunction, the move was postponed indefinitely. Cairo is full of spies and it was essential to give the impression to anyone who came into the hotel on behalf of the opposition to see what was happening with the dolphins, that there was no activity and that preparations appeared to have been disbanded. No activity – no panic to get another injunction. And the name of ZAS had to be as closely guarded as that of Jahbulon is by Freemasons.

Only one or two key people in the hotel were let into the secret. The one television crew was important; we would need to use their hand-held lamp so that we could see to catch the dolphins. John and I must act the part, sitting forlornly in the bar for an hour, bemoaning our bad luck over glasses of beer and helping the word to go round the hotel that we were contemplating flying home empty-handed the following day. With the pool in darkness and the hotel's public rooms fairly empty of people by half an hour after midnight, we would then go to the cabins and start assembling the gear. Everything would be done indoors, quietly, and if it meant breaking a bit of wood off a doorway in order to manhandle through the two dolphin frameworks with their slings when the time came, Monsieur Speck was more than happy to let his carpenter repair the damage the following day. At 2 a.m. on the dot we would emerge from the cabin, meet the television crew and ask them to shine a lamp on the pool. We would catch the animals, grease their skins carefully with the special mixture that my friend Mr Donald, the chemist in Lightwater, makes up for me, settle them in their slings supported by the frameworks, have a shower and then ride off with our patients in a pantechnicon which would be waiting, with its lights off, at the back gate of the hotel. Salem would fix it so that we drove straight out to the aircraft and that men were on hand to load our precious cargo at once. Then, with a bit of luck, it would be chocks away dead on 4.30 a.m., just when the sky began to lighten.

'With such a small team of people in the know,' said John, 'you'll have to come in the water with me and help me catch.' The zoo vet wasn't going to wait, dry and comfortable on the pool-side, for the animals to come to him on this occasion.

'Will it be an underpants job?' he asked. He had seen me so many times go into dolphin or whale pools in my Y-fronts; it has become, I suppose, one of the minor spectacles of the marineland world. But on this occasion he would be disappointed.

'I've brought some jazzy new trunks with blue parrots on them,' I replied solemnly.

In the event, things went more or less according to plan. The television lamp only illuminated a small area of the pool surface, and its reflected glare made seeing the dolphins under water very difficult. But eventually we hauled them out, with me puffing mightily, having imbibed a good half-pint of water. The pantechnicon's engine wouldn't fire, so we had to push-start the enormous vehicle. I puffed the more after that. But then we rattled and banged through the pot-holed streets of the city keeping the dolphins damp with water from plastic flower sprayers. At the airport there was a long pause at customs, and I began to worry that another legal booby trap had been detonated, but no, Salem was there, talking and talking with a fistful of grubby pounds. Presently we rolled across the tarmac to the waiting cargo jet.

Quickly the dolphins were loaded, and their frameworks securely strapped down. They were surrounded by boxes of fresh green beans. Abdel Nasser said good-bye to his 'fish'. He looked rueful at the prospect of his return to the long-suffering ranks of bell-hops later that day. John and I gave him all the Egyptian money we had, which seemed to cheer him up a bit. A photographer and journalist from *Today*, who had somehow ferreted out the fact of our secret departure, had inveigled their way into flying with us. A pretty Egyptian hostess who would look after us during the flight, while we looked after the animals, handed round coffee. Monsieur Speck and his entourage shook hands with everybody and looked like men just reprieved from Death Row. Salem fixed a group photograph with the president of ZAS in the middle holding a large plastic dolphin that had appeared from nowhere. And then, with a clunk, the cargo door closed tight, the engines turned over and at exactly 04.30 hours, ZAS flight 101 was cleared for take-off.

I have never accompanied dolphins on a better flight. Nemo and Limo lay quietly in their slings, whistling occasionally to one another, while John and I took turns to go back, check their skin temperatures, spray them lightly with water, and use crushed ice for cooling the flukes and flippers when necessary. There was, as usual, no need to give them Valium or other tranquillizers, and with the weather good and no turbulence to shake the aircraft, we didn't have to reposition the dolphins in mid-flight. There was time to sleep a little and later eat the breakfast that ZAS had thoughtfully provided for us.

Half an hour ahead of schedule, we landed at Nice. Michael and a crew from Marineland were there, as were the fire brigade with one of their special trucks. The Antibes fire brigade takes a great pride not only in tackling fires, but also in involving itself in anything to do with water – including dolphins. Often in the past they had happily helped transport animals, including killer whales, and would turn out with their hoses at a moment's notice if we had to empty a pool and refill it with fresh water, as I sometimes request when needing to rehydrate a dehydrated animal rapidly. Dolphins can drink through their skins.

Now the firemen carried the two dolphins to their truck. Blue lights, sirens and twenty minutes later, Nemo and Limo were floated out of their slings into the clear blue water of the hospital pool, with four of Marineland's staff in wet suits swimming near them in case they were at first stiff and needed assistance. Their help went uncalled for; both the dolphins shot like arrows through the water, rolling and leaping with effortless grace. I went on to the feeding platform with a bucket of fish and they darted over to me at once. I held a whole herring in each hand, arms stretched out over the pool. The dolphins jumped almost clear of the water, each taking a fish and swallowing it with gusto as they plunged back. Immediately they bobbed up again, mouths open, squawking, asking for more. And I agreed whole-heartedly with what John said when he came over: 'It isn't wishful thinking, David. They look happier here after only five minutes!'

Meanwhile, back in Cairo, Monsieur Linehard's lawyers had, at some point during the last few hours, realized the weakness of obtaining an injunction on a single airline. There was a better way of stopping anyone eloping with the dolphins. At precisely the time when we touched down on French soil, a new injunction was served in Cairo on Monsieur Speck and the Meridien Hotel, preventing them from moving the animals. But of course, by then, the birds – the dolphins – had literally flown. How fortunate it was for Nemo and Limo that the lawyers hadn't thought of that tactic the day before.

The temperaments of the two dolphins did indeed alter dramatically from the moment they arrived in Antibes. No more petulant squeaking or snapping at fingers; they positively beamed good fellowship, played dolphin games and, what pleased me most, grew plump. Their blood analyses stayed abnormal, however – constantly signalling the presence of long-standing infection. They are still under treatment even as I write.

Naturally a great fuss was made of the pair by everyone from the press and television to the French government, who congratulated Marineland on the rescue operation. Brigitte

Bardot, who lives not far away and is now heavily involved in animal welfare matters, promised to arrive at the drop of a hat with an army of like-minded ladies to blockade Marineland's gates should anyone try to take Nemo and Limo back. And the world and his wife wanted to be photographed close to the two lucky *abandonnés*. 'Vive Nemo et Limo!' was shouted over many a pool-side glass of champagne by mayors, beauty queens and reporters who came to see them. From Cairo other things were said. 'Common thieves and kidnappers' John and I were branded, predictably. There were dark murmurings about Interpol. I suppose that, legally, we had indeed wilfully absconded with someone else's property. Thief, then, I must confess to be. But as the arguments continue to rattle back and forth between Monsieur Linehard and the Meridien, and lawyers for Marineland, the hotel and the dolphins' owner hold meetings in Cairo, Marseilles, Paris and Nice, no end to the dispute seems in sight. Watching Nemo and Limo sporting in the Provençal sunlight, I am more convinced than ever that my debut as an international criminal was one of the most worthwhile things I have ever done. I don't feel the shadow of the guillotine falling across me just yet.

5 The Year of the Panda

A bearlike black and white animal that eats copper and iron
lives in the Qionglai Mountains south of Yandao county.
Anonymous, The Classics of Seas and Mountains (770–256 BC)

Chinese astrology gives each year an animal's name – the year
of the dog, rat and so on. There is, however, no year in the
cycle symbolized by that uniquely Chinese beast, the giant
panda. Nevertheless 1986 was for me, without doubt, The
Year of the Panda – and an ill-starred panda at that.

It began with my receiving a thorough pasting from my
young friend Chu-Lin, the panda born in Madrid Zoo after
we had artificially inseminated his mother, Shao-Shao. Chu-
Lin was by now full grown, but still enjoyed romping on the
grass with his two keepers, Mario and Angel. Accustomed
since shortly after his birth to human contact, he was relatively
easy for me to examine. I could go in with him, stroke
him, tickle his ears, prod his stomach, and even take his
temperature when he was napping – something that pandas
do, on and off, for around ten hours a day. Stroking conscious
pandas is a great privilege that is rarely safe even in the few
zoos who possess them, and the feel of the fur is not as soft
and pleasing as you might imagine, but rather harsh and
greasy – a necessary protection in the cool, wet, bamboo
forests.

Although I have many favourite animals (of which frogs
are, I think, my *most* favourite), the giant pandas, particularly
those at the zoo in Madrid, are special to me – not just because
of their great rarity and the thrill and fascination of having
the responsibility for some of them, but mainly because of
their inscrutability, their innate *mystery*. I can often get part
way into the mind of a chimpanzee, elephant or tiger – I know
what he or she is thinking, feeling – but I look into the
rather small dark eyes of a panda and see nothing but my

miniaturized reflection in the pupils. Even when playing together there is a sense of being quietly, orientally, mocked in the way that Chinese people, inheritors of a more ancient culture, often regard those they call *gwailo*, 'foreign devils', Westerners, from behind a mask of impassivity. In the past few years we have learned a great deal about the giant panda, *pi* or *daxiongmao* ('large bear-cat' and 'he who eats copper and iron') as it is known in China. We have found, for example, that it is a rather laid-back individual who travels on average only half a kilometre a day and, besides its beloved bamboo. also eats wild parsnips and waterweed and over a hundred other kinds of plant and sometimes animals like monkeys, deer fawns and rodents – if it's lucky enough to catch one. But I don't know how pandas think – they give even less away than bears, to whom they are only distantly related.

I travelled to Madrid with a television crew from Border Television to film some items for showing on their popular 'Nature Trail' children's programme. We filmed sequences on prairie dogs, tigers, okapis and komodo dragons, and then began the star item on the giant pandas. After de-scaling the teeth of Chang-Chang, the old male, with an ultra-sound machine under light anaesthetic (a procedure that I have to do once or twice a year in order to control the accumulation of tartar deposited by the special sloppy diet he has), we decided that I should present a piece about feeding the pandas and then end up having some fun with young Chu-Lin. I had played a panda version of tag with him before.

Things started to go wrong when I began to talk to camera about bamboo, and how inefficiently the panda digestive system utilizes the stuff. 'Imagine,' I said, 'eating around thirteen kilos of hard, indigestible stems like this every day,' and, ever conscious that television is a visual medium, bit down hard on a thick piece of bamboo to illustrate the point. A flash of agony shot through my mouth – half of an incisor tooth had snapped off!

Tending thereafter to mumble through partly closed lips, I proceeded to the fun and games scene. Out came Chu-Lin on to his grass paddock with its logs, trees, climbing frame and water barrel – great for playing tag around. 'Now Chu-Lin and I will play our favourite game of tag,' I announced as the camera rolled again, trying to smile without opening my mouth, and with my upper jaw throbbing. 'He'll chase me and touch me with one of his forepaws that carry those remarkable extra bamboo-grasping thumbs. Then, I'll chase him.' Oh, what fun, children, was the impression I had to give. Oh, what I'd give for a Distalgesic and a shot of Novocain, was what I was thinking.

I had made the elementary mistake of presuming upon a giant panda, of deciding on tag without first asking him whether tag was the game he felt like playing today. It at once became evident that tag wasn't on the agenda. No, he had in mind another, rougher game – all-in wrestling! The rules were simple; he was sure I'd pick them up straight away. He would grab me with his powerful forelegs, throw me to the ground and then hold one of my arms in his jaws which are as strong and toothy as you'd expect in a bamboo-chomper. When I yelled it would count as a fall. Nothing serious, nothing malevolent about this, you understand – just a new panda game he'd dreamed up during one of those inscrutable frequent naps.

All of this was being filmed from outside the enclosure; the director, camera and sound men were on the other side of the dry moat that stops Chu-Lin going out to play his games with the public. To the television crew everything appeared to be going well. The all-in wrestling, which they hadn't expected, was far more spectacular than the tag which they had.

Of course, while my playmate was going for me with the enthusiasm of Mike Tyson, do not imagine I was just standing there. Not at all. I was doing three things simultaneously: trying to describe in clear, interesting, calmly enunciated English what delightful animals pandas are, children, though (with some emphasis) they are not as *cuddly* as you might think; skipping backwards with one eye on the camera, another eye on the logs, trees *and moat* towards which I was being driven; and brilliantly improvising a countermove that would keep Chu-Lin occupied. This countermove worked quite well at first. I shall call it, as a wrestling commentator might, a Reverse Head Panda Push. I found that if I pressed down on to the top of Chu-Lin's head as he grabbed my knee, he would curl up into a ball, release me, do a forward somersault – and then renew the attack. The television crew thought this first-class entertainment for the kiddies.

But I was tiring fast. The panda consisted of around a hundred kilos of chunky muscle and he just kept on grabbing. He badly wanted that fall, with his teeth holding my arm. Like a child or a puppy who gets over-excited during play and loses a little control, so Chu-Lin was increasing the force of his movements. My strength began literally to drain away and I was breathing hard. The panda's teeth sheared through the leather jacket I was wearing; he was determined to bring me down. I was now in serious trouble, gasping for air and sensing, to my horror, that I would shortly collapse. The Border Television crew continued filming, unaware of my predicament – I was obviously hamming it up a bit – but that was nothing new.

From somewhere in my bowels I gathered enough air to shout '*Mario!*' The keeper, who was standing watching from outside the paddock gate, understood at once. He dashed in and pulled Chu-Lin off me. I have never felt so near to flaking out as at that moment. I was bruised, stiff and exhausted. My friend Chu-Lin had given me a more frightening experience than anything I could remember, even including the elephant at Belle Vue which tried, with malice aforethought, to crush me against a wall with its forehead, or the zebras that hunted me in the reserve at Windsor or the leopard that got his claw hooked into my Achilles tendon. Nowadays I'm quite proud of the patches on the leather jacket that are my souvenirs of Chu-Lin's game!

When we'd finished filming, I went with the television crew to spend a pleasant evening in the old part of the city near the Plaza Mayor, going from bar to bar having *tapas* of *jabugo* ham here and octopus there, accompanied by the red wine of the house. It was when I went into the men's room in the ninth or tenth bar that I thought I saw an unusual tint to my urine, rather like that of rosé wine. But it was so dark in the tiny loo which consisted, typically, of just a hole in the floor flanked by two porcelain foot grips, that I couldn't be sure. When I mentioned the phenomenon to my friends, someone suggested it was the strong, rough wine we'd consumed. It didn't seem likely, but sometimes people do pee red after eating a lot of beetroots. Perhaps the wine of the Plaza Mayor was coloured chemical plonk. It certainly didn't taste like Vega Sicilia.

Back at the hotel I made straight for the bathroom and urinated in the sink so that I could see the colour against the white glaze. No doubt about it. Rosé d'Anjou. I had no pain or frequency. The following morning the colour was still there, but apart from the post-panda stiffness and the sensitive half-tooth, I felt fine. Had Chu-Lin somehow damaged one of my kidneys, I wondered, but when the ruddy tinge disappeared later in the day and I was passing what could be taken for Muscadet, I thought no more about it.

It was in Milan two weeks later, while on one of my regular inspections of north Italian zoos and safari parks, that the colour appeared again. This time it came accompanied by sudden, severe back pain. I flew home at once and an X-ray revealed that Chu-Lin had nothing to do with it; there was a stone like a prickly Heinz bean lodged in my right ureter. It meant an operation and two weeks in hospital; for the first time in my life as a zoo vet I had to take time off work. But there was a phone by the bed to keep in touch with the outside world and I was consoled by two things about the hospital in Windsor: the first person to come to meet me at reception was the chef, who asked me what my preferences were (he turned out to be a master with vegetables); and the prescription of my surgeon, who said I could have gin and tonic or champagne whenever I liked from the time I came round from the anaesthetic (neither of which one fancies at a moment like that – but the thought was cheering).

Not long after I left hospital, Antonio-Luis, my veterinary colleague in Madrid, telephoned with news of Chu-Lin. The animal had, for no apparent reason, begun to drink more than usual. What did I suggest he should do? The first thing was to analyse a sample of urine, looking particularly for evidence of the kidneys leaking protein, and for sugar, the well-known sign of diabetes. Diabetes is quite common in animals and, apart from domestic pets, I'd had cases in camels, wallabies, monkeys and several other species which had, on the whole, been controllable by daily insulin injections and a modified diet, although, except for the monkeys, they hadn't responded to the tablets which are often effective in human patients. It wasn't difficult for Antonio-Luis to obtain the urine sample – he simply sucked some into a syringe from a puddle in Chu-Lin's sleeping quarters. The tests were negative. No sugar, no protein – nothing abnormal about the urine at all.

My friend reported to me each morning on the panda's condition. The thirst progressively increased as time went by; Chu-Lin was soon drinking gallons of water every day, and passing correspondingly vast quantities of urine. Not content with the unlimited, clean, fresh water provided in his quarters, he began to develop an obsession for lapping up any drops of dirty liquid he could find in cracks in the ground or at the grille of a drain. I decided to fly out to give him a thorough examination.

Apart from the excessive drinking, I could find nothing wrong, and the analysis of blood taken after administering a little Valium was that of a normal giant panda. This was puzzling. Perhaps a batch of the special panda flakes, a mixture of cereals and crushed peas imported from England, had somehow been prepared with a surfeit of salt. I had some analysed – it contained the correct amount. Two weeks passed, and Chu-Lin's thirst continued to climb. More ominously, his weight was starting to fall, and he was no longer interested in playing with his stepfather Chang-Chang. Each morning as he left his dormitory and walked down the passageway that leads to the outside paddock, one of his keepers checked his weight by means of the small weighbridge built into the concrete floor. Normally around a hundred kilos, Chu-Lin was steadily losing a few hundred grams a day. Soon, from being merely uninterested in play, the young panda was in a state of unmistakable depression.

To and fro, between London and Madrid, I travelled, sampling anything and everything to do with Chu-Lin, calling in a kidney specialist from the most prestigious private hospital in the city, telephoning London and New York to pick the brains of experts in the obscurest corners of medicine, and trying desperately to find some way of halting the animal's inexorable decline. It was utterly baffling. No clues in the samples. No response to symptomatic drug treatment. I re-read everything I could lay my hands on concerning water balance in the mammal body, on kidney function and diabetes, and came to the conclusion that there must be some sort of leak in Chu-Lin's kidneys, but one which didn't allow protein or anything other than water to escape. Ninety, eighty-five, eighty kilograms; the poor animal began to resemble a bag of bones. He was no longer interested in life, picked gloomily at his food and spent all the time when he wasn't drinking fast asleep.

One of the diseases that I had considered as a possibility was diabetes insipidus, or 'water diabetes', an illness quite unrelated to the commoner diabetes mellitus or 'sugar diabetes' and which (unlike the latter, which is centred in the pancreas) can develop when something goes wrong with part of the pituitary gland beneath the brain. Although never reported previously in pandas, there seemed no reason why it *couldn't* happen to a panda pituitary.

To test the idea, I asked Antonio-Luis to inject Chu-Lin with an extract of pituitary gland prepared for such cases in humans. If the thirst diminished rapidly, I would know I was on the right lines. The injections were given; Chu-Lin seemed at first to consume a little less water, but then, despite repeated doses, returned to drinking like Pantagruel. Antonio-Luis and I were downcast, and when the panda's weight dipped to sixty kilos, I felt the battle was lost. The animal was so weak on his legs that the very act of putting his head down to drink from his bowl was enough to send him crashing forwards. His profound apathy obviated any need for Valium or the special treatment cage, when we were working on him. Desperately I clutched at straws. Herbal preparations – try them. Homoeopathy – why not? There are a few veterinary surgeons using the homoeopathic system in animals in Great Britain. However inexplicable the unorthodox basis of such methods may be, at least it's harmless; and sometimes good results have been obtained in cases where conventional therapy has failed. I contacted a homoeopathic vet who kindly sent me a supply of pills in a little packet bearing the arcane legend LYC 10 M. I did what my colleague instructed, and gave them to Chu-Lin, caring not what esoteric realms I was entering. *Anything*, so long as it might help my panda. It didn't help.

I was still keeping some odd form of diabetes insipidus high on my list of possibilities and so I decided to continue investigations into the panda's pituitary gland. A soft round organ about the size of a grape in a giant panda, it lies in one of the most inaccessible places in the body, at the base of the brain. It is the master gland that exercises control over glands such as the thyroid, ovaries and testes, as well as having its own varied and essential functions. X-rays wouldn't show it up and the surgical approach through the roof of the mouth to inspect it with the naked eye was out of the question. But I badly wanted to look at the pituitary – suppose it had some sort of tumour on it that was causing all the trouble?

There was one machine that could do the job: a CAT scanner, the multi-million dollar contraption that was only to be found in a few of the biggest modern hospitals and which had almost never been used on animals. I say *almost*, for we had received scans of tortoises from California (where else?) which depicted the innards of those most inaccessible difficult-to-diagnose of animals, in startling detail. In the Gulf there was a CAT scanner at a luxury hospital used by the sheikhs who, caring for nothing more than their falcons, apart from themselves, had allowed us full access to any of the departments if we needed it in treating their pets. A Sri Lankan servant with cancer wasn't, of course, given the benefit of such advanced medical wonders, but a falcon and sometimes a gazelle deserved, and *got*, the best; several times I or one of my assistants would march straight into the CAT-scanning department with a chesty peregrine or lame gazelle and the radiographers, radiologists, surgeons and nurses, all of them expatriates, would come running as if it were King Faisal himself having a coronary. In Europe, however, access to CAT scanners was normally impossible for animals, and besides, anything above a certain diameter of torso wouldn't be able to pass through the machine. CAT-scanning elephants and giraffes is out. I reckoned, however, that the scanner could just about cope with a giant panda if his legs were tucked in, and that even a dolphin would be feasible.

For Chu-Lin, then, I needed the use of a CAT scanner. There was only one in Madrid – at a private clinic in the city centre. Dr Cerdan, Director of the Zoo, promised to make representations to the clinic's owners, and if they were agreeable and the Health Ministry gave us permission, I would go to the clinic to see whether we could physically get the panda to and through the big machine.

Things moved quickly; both the clinic and the Ministry gave us the green light. With Antonio-Luis I made a reconnaissance of the clinic. We found that the scanner was on the ground floor, the doors and corridors were wide enough and, crucially, that the circular hole in the centre of the scanner through which Chu-Lin would have to move would *just* take his now emaciated trunk. We would scan him after hours, when the traffic was light and the clinic had finished with its human patients. Everything was arranged for the next night and *two* human ambulances were booked – one to carry Chu-Lin, and the other as back-up in case of emergencies.

Antonio-Luis and I went back to the Casa de Campo and worked out a precise timetable for the operation.

At 9.30 the following evening, our treasure among the bamboos, for that is what Chu-Lin means in Mandarin, was coaxed, supported, almost carried into a large, well-ventilated transport box, which was then put aboard the first ambulance. Antonio-Luis, Liliana his wife, the other veterinarian at the zoo and I travelled with him. Just before we set off I gave the panda a little Valium to minimize any anxiety he might feel during what I thought might be a noisy ride at break-neck speed. How right I was! With two Guardia Civil motor cyclists in front and the reserve ambulance behind, and consequently four sets of sirens and flashing blue lights, we roared out of the zoo and through the wooded parkland of the Casa de Campo. The sound was deafening. The Guardia Civil men were skilled, high-speed drivers, accustomed to carving their way through the often densely clogged traffic of Madrid like hot knives in butter. One would charge ahead to block off junctions, while the other, John Wayne at the head of the Fifth Cavalry, took us straight through the red lights. Luckily, we had roped Chu-Lin's box to the ambulance floor – for at every bend, as the tyres added their screams to the din, my colleagues and I were bounced off the walls of the vehicle like peas in a drum. There was almost a disaster as we crossed Castellana and the driver had to slam on his brakes to miss, by a whisker, a collision with a truck driver who felt that his green light was green, no matter that the *loco* Guardia waving his arms about appeared to think differently. Everything loose in the ambulance, including us, careered forwards, and slammed into a partition. A portable oxygen apparatus smashed through a window, showering glass on our driver. Now I understood why Dr Cerdan had insisted on the second ambulance, and Antonio-Luis half-jokingly remarked that it was an oversight not to have taken Valium ourselves.

At last, thank God, we arrived at the clinic. Before unloading Chu-Lin we gave him an injection of light anaesthetic and, when he was sleeping, brought him out of the box on to one of the clinic's operating-theatre trolleys. Then the panda was whisked down the corridors to the CAT scanner department, where radiologists were already sitting before banks of computer screens in a side room. Even in his skeletal state, Chu-Lin had the frame of a dumpy, thick-set individual. To go through the doughnut-like ring of the machine meant slimming him further, by trussing his legs tight into his trunk. Three canvas straps soon had the unconscious animal looking like a rather hairy roll of butcher's meat. Gently we laid him on the moving slide that would pass him, in precisely controlled jerks, through the scanner's centre. As it was the pituitary gland in which I was principally interested, I asked for computer images to be taken and filmed every millimetre from the tip of his nose to the top of his neck. From then on one-centimetre 'slices' of the rest of his body would do nicely.

Nervously, for Antonio-Luis and I are always on tenter-hooks when the pandas are under anaesthetic, we watched as the machine was switched on and Chu-Lin began to disappear, nose-tip first, into the scanner. If anything went wrong, I couldn't do much until he came out at the other side. The computer screens began to display cross-sections of his head. Showing soft tissue as well as bone, scanning pictures are far more detailed and revealing than X-rays. As the minutes passed, a succession of images, resembling I thought the cut surface of one of those continental pâtés that contain chunks of truffle, meat and olives, came up on the fluorescent screens and was stored in the computer memory. For the first time ever, a live giant panda's whole anatomy was being looked at. Here was the brain with its various parts, the delicate mechanisms of the inner ear, there the heart, the liver, the kidneys – we watched the procession of pictures that illustrated a *whole* animal composed of organs, tissues, liquids, gases, fragile membranes, solid gristle, soft fat and dense bone, quite unlike the ghostly shadows captured by X-rays. During the scan there was no time to study individual images; that would have to wait till later.

At last, after almost an hour, the amazing machine spewed

forth our panda and he was taken back, already blinking and licking his lips, to the waiting ambulance. Again the Ride of the Valkyries would have seemed like a leisurely evening promenade in comparison to our furious convoy as it recrossed the city streets and avenues to take this most illustrious of out-patients home. By midnight Chu-Lin was back at his bowl, drinking water as avidly as the fairytale frog that made the fountain run dry.

The films of the computer images arrived at the zoo the next morning and we studied them carefully. It was like poring over an anatomy textbook with hundreds of illustrations, each one slightly different from the next. What I knew about the panda's insides had been gleaned from a relatively small number of sources – the first descriptions by the famous Père David (of Père David deer fame) in 1870 that had so excited the French scientific world, and the careful dissection of Chi-Chi performed by London Zoo when that most popular of pandas died in 1972, after fourteen years at Regent's Park. I had photographs and measurements of Chi-Chi's pituitary gland. When our scans came to the part of the head (a pit called the sella turcica) where the pituitary gland should have been safely ensconced, we could find nothing that we could identify as the gland itself. Although this was the first panda scan, the basic anatomy was clearly identifiable, but neither we, nor radiologists we consulted, could say, hand on heart, that such and such a blob on the film was the pituitary. All mammals have pituitaries. We know pandas have them. You and I, and pigs and elephants, can't live without a pituitary. Nor, we are certain, can a giant panda. The mystery of Chu-Lin's 'missing pituitary' has not so far been solved. It might seem tempting to theorize that his had withered to a mere husk and so caused the disease. I don't believe it, and prefer the explanation that our interpretation of the scans is in some way imperfect.

We had CAT-scanned Chu-Lin and learned much, but nothing that could help improve the odds against him. What now? Every day I was continuing to read anything I could find about 'water diabetes' and associated matters. We were given the animal herbal 'kidney injections' and had begun considering using the curious, and very Spanish, alternative medicine technique of taking a little blood from the patient and then at once re-injecting it under the skin. Again, it sounded crazy, but it was harmless, and some Spanish doctors swore by it for humans.

One evening, I was sitting in the cramped little study of my home in Lightwater, reading a paper on treating certain types of 'water diabetes' in humans. I came across a reference to the value, in some instances, of giving diuretic drugs.

Now, diuretic drugs make people (and animals) pass *more* urine than normal and the one thing I would have given my eye teeth for was to have Chu-Lin passing *less* and drinking *less*. A lot less. But the article referred to the 'paradoxical' effect of the diuretic in treating the disease – no one was sure how, but it did the *opposite* of what you might imagine.

I, like most vets, was familiar with the family of diuretic drugs mentioned, the thiazides. They were used in evacuating accumulations of fluid in heart disease and certain dropsies. Nowadays I mainly use them for reducing soggy swellings on the underbelly of elephants.

I telephoned Antonio-Luis straight away. 'I know it sounds *tonto*,' I explained, 'but I would like you to give Chu-Lin some Saluric.'

Mario, the younger of the two panda-keepers at Madrid, was on the night shift; he and Angel were maintaining a round-the-clock watch in the panda house. As instructed, he had given one of the diuretic tablets to Chu-Lin at midnight, after crushing and mixing it with a little honey and yoghurt. Coaxing the panda to eat anything by this stage was very difficult. Mario wondered what the latest in the interminable line of potions prescribed by the *veterinarios* was supposed to do; he himself was sure that the end was near. It was just a question of when. He hoped it was while Angel was on duty.

Bright morning light streamed in through the windows of

the panda kitchen. It was the best time of day in the zoo. The animals had the great gardens to themselves for an hour or two of daylight. Mario could hear them announcing, in their various ways, that they had awakened – the distant yawn-snarl of a lion, capuchins twittering like birds and rousing sleepy ducks who had spent the night hauled out on the monkeys' island, the clatter of pelican bills as the birds waddled, like a team of animal inspectors, round the pathway stopping briefly, as is their wont, to stare at each paddock or pond before moving on. Soon Angel would arrive to relieve him; it was time to prepare the pandas' breakfast. Into a stainless steel bowl the keeper measured the usual ingredients – five spoons of soya, one spoon of honey, olive oil, invalid food, dried yeast, vitamin mixture and 300 grams of panda flakes. He added some hot water and mixed the lot thoroughly into a porridge. That, together with some fine branches of bamboo, would start off Chang-Chang's day. Into Chu-Lin's bowl he put a carton of yogurt and a spoon of boiled rice; if he were lucky the dying panda would lap up half of it, very, very slowly, before turning his head away.

Mario went down the corridor, opened the door to Chang-Chang's quarters and went in. '*Buenos dias, viejo,*' he greeted the old male, still lying comfortably on his sleeping shelf, and put down the bowl. Chang-Chang would descend and eat it in his own good time. Mario went on to the next massive wooden door – Chu-Lin's. He put one eye to the peep-hole. 'Perhaps today is the day,' he thought, steeling himself as he had for the past month, ready for the last act in the tragedy. This time, however, he couldn't see anything through the fish-eye peep-hole. Strange. It was blocked. Then he understood, he saw. An eye was pressed against the other side of the peep-hole, *trying to look at him*! Quickly Mario slid the bolts and swung open the door. Wobbly, very wobbly, there stood Chu-Lin looking up at him – at the bowl! *Chu-Lin wanted his breakfast!* Normally there would be signs that the panda had passed torrents of urine during the night. Mario looked at the floor – dry everywhere. *Chu-Lin hadn't peed!* His hands trembling with excitement, Mario bent down and placed the bowl in front of the panda; almost, but not quite, losing his balance, Chu-Lin lowered his head and sucked up the yoghurt and rice – every drop of it. Forgetting to close the door behind him, Mario dashed back to the kitchen and grabbed the telephone. While he was telling the incredible news to Antonio-Luis, Chu-Lin wobbled into the kitchen and began sniffing at a bag of panda flakes. '*Un milagro, un milagro!*' shouted the keeper down the phone. 'It's a miracle!' Which it was.

The two keepers (Mario refused to go home at the end of his shift) watched Chu-Lin all that day. He drank water, but only a normal amount, and he ate his food, even a few bamboo leaves, with more interest than of late, though not with gusto. I need hardly describe how ecstatic I was after taking the daily phone call from Madrid at the unusually early hour of seven o'clock, nor that, after arranging to press on with the diuretic regime, I opened a bottle of champagne for my breakfast.

Two tablets a day did the trick. A week passed, and still the thirst did not reappear. The panda's appetite grew stronger and soon the needle on the scales began to move up at his daily weigh-ins. The long slow haul to recovery had begun, and we experimented to discover the lowest dose of the Saluric tablets that would suffice to keep Chu-Lin on course. It seemed to be about half a tablet each morning. After a month he had gained seven kilos and was much stronger on his legs. Another month and he was at eighty-five kilos, and showed the first signs of wanting to play again with his stepfather. Slowly I reduced the dose of the Saluric to a quarter and then to an eighth of a tablet. Eventually I stopped them altogether. Nothing untoward happened. Chu-Lin was a plump, hundred-kilo, chirpy giant panda again and the crowds of Spanish children could come, as they had before, to chant, 'Chu-Lin, Chu-Lin, Chu-Lin!' to the most famous animal in Madrid as he sat contentedly in the shade of a tree with his back against the trunk and his paws resting on his paunch. His strange illness has never been fully explained, nor has it so far recurred. Just to see him there, giving an audience to his admirers, is enough for me.

The next panda poser in that Year of The Giant Panda involved Chang-Chang (the name means 'strong') Chu-Lin's stepfather and long-suffering playmate. As soon as I met him, after he'd arrived as a gift from the Chinese government to King Juan Carlos, I suspected that he was, in human terms, in early middle age. Pandas are thought to live for about thirty years, and the more opportunities I had to examine him as the years went by, the more signs of 'senior panda citizenship' I recognized – his teeth, figure, coat colour all indicated that he hadn't been a brand-new model when he left Peking on his journey of embassy to the Spanish court. (The King has a palace not far from the zoo where the panda house had been built ready for Chang-Chang and his mate Shao-Shao.)

In 1986, however, I noticed something more ominous than greying hairs when I was giving him a routine medical check-up. Barely visible to the naked eye, a small, oblong, smoke-coloured patch had developed in the centre of the transparent cornea of each eye. Chang-Chang was totally untroubled by their presence, and there was no sign of inflammation associated with them. Through the powerful lens of an ophthalmoscope I saw that the patches were composed of minute globules of some liquid, probably a kind of fat called lipid, lying within the eyes' window. Such degenerative changes generally occur in old age in dogs and human beings; like wrinkles, they are inscriptions of the moving finger of time and could perhaps only be tackled, if they became very dense and extensive, by means of a corneal transplant. Panda transplant donors, are, of course, as easily found as the Philosopher's Stone. But I was certain that the patches were of a size and in a position that would not interfere with vision. Doctor Barnett, the veterinary ophthalmologist who has done some fine cataract operations for us on exotic animals (including the first-ever in Europe on a sea lion) agreed, when I described Chang-Chang's condition, that nothing should be done except regular eye checks. (No, *not* with one of those optician's charts where you have to read off a line of letters – anyway, pandas would need a chart with Chinese characters rather than the Roman alphabet!)

Many months passed and then, one day, Antonio-Luis, making one of his regular telephone calls, reported that Chang-Chang's eyes had gone much worse overnight. The left eye looked blue-white from a distance, and there was also a white spot in the centre of the right eye. More alarmingly, the panda was sometimes bumping into things as he walked around. That afternoon found me, as so often, on the British Airways Madrid flight.

The old boy wasn't too difficult to examine, and I didn't need my instruments to see that the left eye was badly ulcerated all around the lipid patch. Erosions and white blotches were blocking and distorting the passage of light. A similar process was starting in the other eye. I was appalled. To have lost the over-thirsty Chu-Lin would have been a major tragedy; for Chang-Chang to go blind would be almost as bad.

'Get me the best ophthalmic surgeon in Madrid – we'll tranquillize Chang-Chang tomorrow morning,' I said to Antonio-Luis – and lo, it was done. The following day a beautiful, green-eyed lady, Dr Pilar, drove into the zoo – I had the expertise I needed.

Eye injuries and diseases of many kinds are not uncommon in exotic animals. Elsewhere I have described replacing the dislocated eye of a Père David deer in a storm; and cataracts in orphan animals caused by artificial foods that contained too much, or the wrong sort of, sugar caused me many headaches when I was a young zoo vet. In 1976 in a BBC television 'World About Us' programme depicting my work, I removed the eye of an alligator; and I have often been called in to amputate the chronically swollen 'third eyelid' of a lion or tiger. But the animal called *Homo sapiens* is heir to more of the degenerative type of diseases than many of my patients, because it lives for longer than most of them and abuses itself so persistently with alcohol, tobacco leaves, curious diets and other things. Medical doctors tend therefore to see a higher proportion of chronic degenerative pathology than veterinary surgeons who in turn, see more acute pathology than their medical colleagues. That is why I valued the opinion of the good Dr Pilar; and as disease processes in all mammals, including man and giant pandas, are essentially the same, it mattered not that she had never before squinted into the eyes of anybody like Chang-Chang.

Yes, it was a degeneration and the sudden flare-up was a secondary infection, the ophthalmologist opined. No, blindness need not follow if we moved quickly, and no, surgery was not indicated. I touched the tip of a sterile swab gently against the cornea of the tranquillized panda's right eye and repeated the procedure for the left. The swabs went with Dr Pilar back to her clinic. Three days later she telephoned. The germ that had invaded the lipid patches in Chang-Chang's eyes had been identified. Its name was *Pseudomonas*, and it was sensitive to an antibiotic called gentamycin. We would have to apply some gentamycin to Chang-Chang's eyes four times a day, and obviously couldn't dope him every time in order to do it. Chang-Chang is not as friendly a character as Chu-Lin and it would have been very dangerous to take liberties, such as poking tubes or droppers close to the eye, with him. He does love sweet apples, however, and I devised a method of introducing the gentamycin drops simply and safely, both for the animal and ourselves.

His outdoor paddock is divided into two by a wire mesh fence. With him on one side and us on the other, he could be tempted up to the mesh by a supply of juicy red fruit. While, say, Antonio-Luis pushed a chunk of apple through the fence, I would squirt the antibiotic liquid into his eye from an ordinary hypodermic syringe and needle held about half a metre away from his head. Though gentamycin solution doesn't sting, Chang-Chang didn't appreciate being zonked at regular intervals by some supposedly adult vet who retained an infantile delight in water pistols, but his passion for apples transcends such provocations. Grumbling gently he literally turned the other cheek – which conveniently allowed me to squirt him in the second eye!

Chang-Chang's eyes improved dramatically, he stopped walking into trees and door frames, and after ten days of the apple and squirt treatment he was back to normal, but still, of course, with the original, oblong, lipid patches in his corneas. If they ever flare up again we'll start the same treatment at once. 1986 came to a close without any further panda alarums.

6 Full-flavoured Cuba

The Sharke, or Tiberune, is a Fish like vnto those which we call Dog-fishes, but that he is farre greater.
Sir Richard Hawkins, *Observations in His Voyage Into the South Sea*

'Doctor, we must hurry. A young man, a neighbour of mine, has been injured!' My companion, a bespectacled Cuban with black walrus moustache and snow-white teeth that were permanently on show, hustled me out of the once-grand house that serves now as a headquarters of the government trading bureau, and towards the battered Lada that waited at the kerb, chugging unhealthily.

'But why me? Surely the hospital services . . .' I said as we juddered over the pot-holes through the pleasant suburb of Miramar with its wide avenues, stands of royal palms (*Roystonea regia*), spick and span embassies, crumbling villas, smart American-style motorbike policemen in blue uniforms at the road junctions, and knots of schoolchildren wearing red neckerchiefs, on their way to school.

'The doctors have seen him. But he is a special case. Your sort of case, *compañero* – he's been stung by a fish. And besides, his mother is very worried. It's his wedding next week.'

Jorge said no more as we made our way along the Malecon, the Havana sea-wall, towards the old Spanish Morro fortress and lighthouse that overlooks the narrow harbour entrance. Going through the tunnel bored beneath the inlet we ran into the flat countryside to the east of the city.

It was 1986 and I was on the second of a series of visits I would make to Cuba. Since the late 1970s, the number of successful dolphin births in European marinelands had risen steadily, along with the life expectancy of these animals, as standards of pool design, water treatment and health care had improved by leaps and bounds. We had learnt much about cetaceans since those early days in 1968 when I'd gone to the

US Navy's Undersea Warfare Division at Point Magu in California to learn the basic techniques of handling these unique animals. Losses of dolphins from epidemic disease like swine erysipelas, or because water was under-filtered or over-treated chemically, no longer happened. Cheapjack summer season and travelling dolphin shows with small portable pools have virtually disappeared in Europe, and there was a welcome framework of national and international regulations developing to oversee the welfare of captive marine mammals.

The total number of dolphins taken from the sea by *all* the world's marinelands in 1986 was less than forty, fewer than were being bred in the marinelands, and a minute fraction of the thousands that died, and still die, every year in the nets of tuna fleets or with their throats cut by Japanese fishermen. But these few animals, taken under inter-governmental licence, and of a species that was not endangered, were needed for the occasional new marineland that was being constructed, to replace individuals dying from old age or disease, and to bring new blood into breeding groups. We had reached the stage where three generations of marineland-born animals were living happily in some of the big facilities in the United States.

Traditionally, bottle-nosed dolphins had been obtained from American waters in Florida or the Gulf of Mexico. In 1986 I decided to explore another potential source, Cuba. I was attracted by several factors. The shallow coastal waters of that biggest of Caribbean islands are rich in dolphins, manatees and fish and, compared with the tourist-infested US coastline, a few score miles to the north, almost completely unpolluted. With few of the pleasurecraft, water-skiers and speedboats that create noise as well as chemical pollution, and little sewage or chemical effluent being discharged, Miami-fashion, into the ocean, the fauna of Cuban waters comprises species that are no longer to be found near the American seaboard. Clean seas promised clean, healthy dolphins. The Cubans, hungry for hard currency, could offer cheap and efficient air transport to Europe and, significantly, this would mean in most cases a faster journey, pool to pool, for the animals. Jet flights between Havana and European capital cities are frequent and take around nine hours non-stop.

On my first visit to Cuba, a month before, I had instantly fallen in love with the place and its people. There was none of the oppressive police state ambiance that I had imagined, but immigration and customs officials who smiled and joked – can you imagine their US counterparts doing that? – and men and women of every colour from blonde to blue-black with temperaments that blended the laid-back good humour of the West Indies, the Latin passion of Castile and the innate rhythms of Africa and South America. Okay, so they're not the most efficient of folk, and their society is woefully short of many things that we take for granted, among them basic materials. More important is the fact that they are a *loving* people. You may wait, drumming your fingers on the counter, while the abundant staff behind the reception desk greet one another, exchange kisses and giggle over a smidgin of gossip, but you can't be angry with them. Human relations come first with Cubans. Cold communist dogma and bureaucracy hasn't touched the hip-swing of pretty mulatto girls, the cheeky honking of the boys who drive past them in the street, the love of *Salsa*, the dance, and the pride, found since the revolution, not only in *conquistador* blood but also in that of the African slave and the Carib Indian.

True, the island needs a giant DIY store to supply millions of gallons of paint and plaster. The walls of the beautiful town-houses peel and flake, fallen tiles lie unreplaced and antique wooden doors moulder and split. The shops are shabby and have little to sell, the supply of beer is erratic, jeans and trainers draw envious eyes, air-conditioning units work fifty per cent of the time, it's almost impossible to find a photocopier, and a letter to England can take six months to arrive. By democratic standards the Cubans are not a free people, but they are free of grinding poverty (you'll find more beggars round Waterloo Station than in the whole of Havana) and of the diseases of poverty, and they're free of American suzerainty. Education and medical services are of a high standard and widely available to all, there's plenty of excellent rum and fine cigars at cheap prices, you can walk through the back alleys of the inner city without coming to any harm, you can hire a car and drive anywhere in the country without need of permits, and the beaches are among the best in the world. Enough of the travel brochure!

Having selected a pair of dolphins on my previous visit and given them a clean bill of health, I was now in Havana preparing to travel back with them to Madrid. It took time. With no aluminium tubing, fibreglass or plastic sheeting to be had for the construction of strong, light frames in which to suspend the dolphins' travelling hammocks, massive old-fashioned 'coffins' of wood were the only answer. That meant arranging for the university joinery department, situated outside Havana, to start sawing and mortising according to my diagrams. The offices of Cubana, the national airline, had to be visited time after time to book spaces for the animals and their attendants, to ensure that two seats nearest to the galley on the old Ilyushin jets would be reserved for a Cuban vet, Dr José-Manuel Fernandez, and myself, so that we could go down through the trapdoor in the floor of the aircraft at twenty-minute intervals during the flight to check on the dolphins in the cargo hold. I had to negotiate the minimum loading time, so that we could arrive at José Marti Airport at the last possible moment before the aircraft took off, thus reducing the time that the dolphins were out of the water.

Airlines in the USA and Europe, much to my annoyance, often insist on livestock being at the airport two or three hours before departure time. In the Cuban system, where the Aquarium, the Academy of Sciences, the Trading Department and the Airline are all arms of the government, I found that it was possible to bend the rules by persistent talking. My argument ran thus: 'I'll sign the document releasing my client's money to you, the Trading Department, *if* I can have the full co-operation of the Aquarium in providing a fast well-sprung lorry and lots of men to lift the animals in their heavy boxes and *if* the Airline will let me and the dolphins arrive on the tarmac when all the passengers are on board and the flight is ready to go, so that they can be loaded straightaway, the doors closed and the engines started. To help keep the animals cool I must have a night flight, the flight engineer must be willing to adjust the cargo temperature as I instruct him and the animals must be loaded into a position so that they are first off when we arrive at our destination. All these things are possible in the United States, and I would hope that Cuba could do as well – if not better.' With no one wanting to be accused of lacking revolutionary fervour (the island is festooned with hoardings, placards and flags proclaiming things like 'Commander Fidel says Forward with the Revolution' and 'We're all working alongside Fidel and the Party'), I have observed that capitalist individuals from the West tend to get their own way over such matters.

It was essential also, to go to the airport and find the glamorous female army major in chic khaki blouse, contrasting scarf and full make-up, very Israeli I've always thought, who would give me a permit and a squaddie to accompany me while I went to measure the cargo hold and loading door of an aircraft of the appropriate type. Usually this resulted in me then returning to the university carpenters, and asking them to start chopping inches and corners off the dolphin boxes. The problem seems to be either that the Cubans never understand my diagrams despite their protestations of '*Si, Excellente!*' or that no two Russian aircraft come in exactly the same dimensions.

At the Aquarium, whose director is Professor Dario Guitart, a delightful, humane and cultured man who is one of the world's great experts on sharks, and where Che Guevara's daughter is a junior vet, there were other matters to sort out. The place bristles with staff, provides guests like me with generous hospitality in the form of mountains of fried Caribbean fish and devastating Blue Dolphin daiquiri cocktails, but has no equipment. The laboratory exists but is furnished with nothing but some dusty test-tubes and flasks. My final blood samples before the journey, needed to ensure that the animals are one hundred per cent fit to travel, had to be sent to a city hospital. I would receive the results two days later. There were the injections of praziquantel to be given to rid the animals of the curious *Nasitrema* parasitic flukes that commonly live in the blowholes of wild dolphins and which can cause chronic sinusitis.

After all that, there was time to do other things. Like going to see 'the man stung by a fish'.

We arrived at the village where the man lived, a collection of sun-bleached, tired-looking houses with small, earth-floored backyards, foraging poultry and sleepy dogs, and clumps of lemon, tamarind, mammee and custard-apple trees. Jorge led me through a labyrinth of cool pathways between buildings and in through the back door of a house, against the frame of which a number of small cages containing peeping tropical finches were suspended on nails. Like most of the Cuban houses I have seen, the interior was sparsely furnished with long-dull paintwork and faded wallpaper. Sitting on a chair by the window was 'my patient', a young fellow of perhaps twenty-five years of age. He was wearing a shirt and under-pants, and his left leg was propped up on a stool in front of him. 'Miguel, I have brought the English professor,' said Jorge after we had been introduced and shaken hands. 'He will resolve the trouble with your leg.' The trouble with Jorge's leg was plain for all to see; the limb was swollen and an angry red-brown in colour from half-way up the shin almost to the groin. On the front of the shin, close to the lower border of the inflamed area, was a black scab about three centimetres long, surrounded by a narrow zone of purple flaking skin. I bent down and gently touched the leg; it was unnaturally hard and hot. 'The fish did that,' said Miguel. 'I was crossing the river near here, taking a short cut, close to the place where it enters the sea. It is very shallow and I waded across. I must have stood on the fish – it stung me. The pain is not so bad as it was. But the leg is solid. I can't bend the knee.'

'The doctors at the hospital . . .' I replied. 'They have given you treatment which I am sure is the best.'

'*Si, si,*' interrupted Jorge, 'but you, Doctor, are an expert in these marine animals, they say. That is why we want *you* to advise Miguel.' At that moment a small fat woman entered the room, carrying a tray with cups of coffee. '*Professor,* thank you for coming to see my son!' she said at once. 'The problem is the wedding. Miguel is to be married in one week. What are we going to do?'

Miguel had obviously trodden inadvertently on a stingray, perhaps one of the marine forms that often enter estuaries or else the very dangerous South American freshwater stingray which lives in rivers such as the Amazon. I hadn't a clue as to whether such a beast occurred as far north as Cuba. The salt-water kind were, however, abundant in these waters and I'd been out dolphin-catching in Florida when the skipper of the boat I was on, a tough character of Indian extraction, had been stung by a ray we'd pulled in with the nets, and the agony he'd gone through had left a lasting impression on me. Stand on a ray, and it whips up its tail, unsheathing a sharp, dagger-like spine made of bony material and with a toothed and grooved blade. The grooves are lined by a soft, spongy, greyish tissue that produces venom. This venom, to which there is no antidote, produces severe pain and, in some cases, a drop in blood pressure, vomiting, muscular paralysis and death. The serrated edge of the spine inflicts tissue damage where it strikes, and even more when the victim, not unnaturally, withdraws it.

'The wedding, *señora,* I don't quite understand,' I said sipping the strong black coffee. 'With the pain subsiding, the swelling will now gradually reduce, and your son will walk as well as ever. There will, for sure, be no permanent damage to the leg.'

'*Professor!* it isn't the *leg* that concerns me, it's his . . . his . . . *testiculos.* To put it bluntly – *perdoneme, señor* – the old women in the village say that he will not be able to consummate the marriage! What a scandal that would be!'

All eyes were looking at me. 'Well,' I said, 'well . . . the . . . er . . . inflammation of the leg, the stiffness, the pain may – how shall I put it? – make Miguel's performance a little less *vigoroso* than one might have hoped, but . . . but, you can rest assured that eventually . . .'

'*Profesor! Por favor,*' the mother shook her head at me, 'forget the leg – will his *testiculos* be okay after this fish sting?'

'Why, of course, *señora*, there's no way in which this sting —' I had mentally measured the distance between the top border of the now static area of swelling and the young man's private parts, and reckoned it to be a good four inches '— no way in which this sting will affect the function of Miguel's . . . er . . . equipment.'

The woman's round face was at once transformed. She beamed like a golden cherub in a baroque chapel, rushed over and kissed her son and then came to embrace and kiss me. Finally, she darted to the house door and stood in the threshold. Twice, at the top of her voice, she yelled so that the neighbours couldn't have avoided hearing through their open windows. '*Oye! The English professor says Miguel's balls are okay!*' She used the rather vulgar word '*cojones*'. And that was the end of my consultation. Two of the neighbours promptly appeared, carrying bottles of añejo dark rum to share in the family's rejoicing, and there was much patting of backs, and toasts to the leg and other parts of the anatomy of the patient.

'I knew you'd solve the problem,' said Jorge, as we drove back to the city, its buildings of white coral limestone smouldering in the evening sunshine. 'Doctors are all very well for run of the mill complaints, but when it comes to strange things that live in the sea, they don't know nothing.' I said nothing. D C Taylor, Stingray Sting Specialist cum Marriage Counsellor, was savouring the afterglow of the añejo rum.

The flying of the dolphins to Spain was essentially the same as the many other transports that I had taken part in over the previous eighteen years. Originally we had greased the dolphins heavily, and sprayed them continuously using a system of perforated plastic pipes and an electric bilge pump powered by twelve-volt batteries. This technique, which recirculated the water, needed constant supervision to stop the sprayholes becoming blocked by particles of solid excrement. Later we came to regard it as a health risk in the way that it produced a mist of contaminated water that could be inhaled by the dolphin and might theoretically lead to lung infections.

Carrying the animals floating in sea water in waterproof boxes had been tried and found to be disastrous. One dolphin plus water plus box could weigh over half a tonne. It was heavy to lift and move about, cripplingly expensive with air freight being calculated in dollars per pound, and prone to swill the animals around, banging them against the walls of the box, when bad weather was encountered. Worst of all was the tendency of the water to run over the sides of the box when the aircraft banked, or on take-off and landing. Salt water and metal make an unhappy mixture and, after an episode in the late 1960s, when an American jet had to land under manual control because its underfloor electronics had been attacked by salt water leaking from a dolphin box (the aircraft subsequently needed to go in for a complete strip-down to determine the extent of the corrosion), no more salt-water dolphin transports were attempted. Nowadays, the dolphins lie in their padded hammocks, lightly anointed with Vaseline, lanolin or ladies' cold cream over their bodies to keep the skin from drying out; we use a plastic spray from time to time merely to keep them damp, and ice cubes to cool the flippers and the tail. With this technique, a few litres of water in a can and a sack of ice is all we need for a transatlantic flight.

And that is the way I attended to the Cuban dolphins, having remembered to bring to Havana a couple of small plant-sprayers from my local garden centre in Windlesham. Cuba is rich in tropical plant life, but seemingly devoid of such bourgeois things as garden centres and plant-sprayers.

There's just enough space in the cargo hold of an Ilyushin IL-62 to take a maximum of three of the heavy Cuban dolphin 'coffins'. It's well lit, pressurized and the temperature can be held at a desirable sixteen degrees Celsius if one speaks nicely to the flight engineer. The entrance is down a ladder, reached by lifting a trapdoor in the floor of the galley amidships. For the human passengers, a long flight on one of these rather primitive, uncomfortable Russian aircraft, with no film or music provided, and abysmal food, is an ordeal made bearable only by the comparatively cheap prices; I much prefer to sit on a pile of mail bags near the dolphins down below, listening to them squeak to one another, and to me if I whistle in just the right way, with regular supplies of rum and coffee brought down by one of the ever-cheerful cabin staff.

In more than a hundred trans-oceanic flights with dolphins during the past twenty years I haven't lost a single animal in transit nor had a serious in-flight emergency. I've had to use tranquillizers on only two occasions, both during periods of heavy turbulence and, although I carry with me The Bag containing its powerful heart and respiration stimulants, its sedatives and anti-stress drugs, its antibiotics and painkillers, the majority of the bottles have to be thrown away unopened when their expiry date is reached. Travelling with dolphins is almost becoming boring.

In 1987, on one of my Cuban visits, I was planning the transportation of a different kind of marine animal: sharks. Few people are not fascinated by these remarkable fish, many of them (and there are around three hundred species known) anatomically unchanged for a hundred and eighty million years. Although the two biggest fish in the world are sharks – and totally harmless to us – it is the eighteen really dangerous species, the potential man-eaters that stir us. The difficulties of catching, transporting and maintaining such beasts in an aquarium far outweigh those involved with dolphins or whales, but gradually more and more exhibitions of large, live sharks are being successfully set up.

Robert Bennett, my friend and the director of Marineland in Majorca, wanted to create just such a shark display. It is

easy to obtain small sharks or youngsters only a few centimetres long, and most of them will grow quite quickly in the
correct environment, but visitors to an aquarium's shark tank
expect, if not a ten-metre-long great white 'Jaws', at least an
impressive, reasonably big fish that *looks* capable of tearing
chunks off people. Catching large sharks and keeping them
alive during transport is a formidable task.

First you must catch your shark using a hollow hook through
which, down a tube attached to the metal trace, a solution of
fish anaesthetic (often the same chemical that is contained in
sore throat lozenges) is injected. The anaesthetic mixes with
the water in the shark's mouth, flows out through its gills and
is there absorbed, with luck rendering the animal dopey, if
not unconscious. Out of water sharks can be as dangerous as
in it; they can snap those fearsome jaws unexpectedly, hurl
their bodies about and thrash their tails to inflict nasty
wounds, for their skin is covered with thousands of tiny, *but
real*, teeth. Putting them in sea-water containers is not enough
for most species; they need oxygenated water to run through
their gill systems just as if they were swimming forwards. The
movements of their muscular bodies, packed with gristle but
not a single scrap of bone, can quickly fracture wooden and
plastic boxes.

Robert and I resolved to see if we could bring some big
sharks from Cuba on the same aircraft that I had used for the
dolphins. We went to Havana to discuss the possibility with
Professor Guitart at the Aquarium where there are several
species of shark on view, including a tankful of nurse sharks,
some almost two metres long. It was Cuban Mothers' Day,
14 May, when we arrived, and everyone was wearing roses in
honour of their mothers, red ones if they were alive and white
ones if they were dead. Over the usual fried fish and Blue
Dolphin cocktails Robert and I listened as Guitart explained
what would be necessary. 'Try nurse sharks first, before
moving on to the leopard or tiger sharks,' he said; 'they're
tougher, less demanding of oxygen, and they look spectacular,
particularly when feeding.' He took us over to the nurse shark

tank, set on the edge of the sea. The water had been drained out except for a few inches, just deep enough to cover the gills of the large brown sharks with ghoulish white eyes that lay on the bottom. They seemed placid enough, unprotesting as two men walked among them in bare feet brushing the tank floors and walls to remove encrustations of algae. Pushed out of the way with a man's foot, they behaved as amenably as tame sheep; however nurse sharks, though not the most dangerous of species, have been known to attack human beings.

'Normally we send only small sharks by air, in plastic bags containing a little sea water and inflated with air before sealing,' said the Professor, as he climbed down into the tank with the sharks and stroked the biggest one along its back. 'We have no experience with the transporting of large ones. Do you have any ideas?'

'I was thinking perhaps of a long, shallow, watertight box with a dry compartment for a battery at one end,' I said. 'The shark would lie half-submerged, and a pump would circulate water from its head backwards; a built-in sprinkler would provide aeration.'

'The box would have to be sealed with a lid – perhaps a transparent one – and you'd have to stop the fish thrashing.'

'How do you suggest we do that – tranquillizer in the water?'

'No – fix it firmly but gently with arched wooden dividers in the box, shaped to the shark's body contours and padded with rubber.' We drew up some sketches. It *looked* a good idea – but would it work in practice, and keep the animal alive for a period of a little over twelve hours until it arrived in Majorca?

'Let's try an experiment,' I suggested. 'Take the measurements of one of your biggest sharks, make a box and put it on a truck and trundle it around Havana for half a day to see if the method is feasible.' Guitart agreed and Robert and I, armed with a tape measure, descended into the drained tank. Paddling about with our bare ankles touching twenty-centimetre broad mouths armed with rows of thorny teeth was a new experience for me. It was impossible to imagine what the sharks might be thinking, and quite unlike doing the same thing with dolphins. Once in a while a dolphin might playfully nip your leg, but it was rare for them to draw blood, and I've never seen a significant bite inflicted by a dolphin on a human being, even when annoyed. The worst, only a small cut on the knee, was endured by Rob Heyland, the actor who played me in the 'One By One' television series, when we were filming in France.

Taking the length, width and height of the sharks proved no problem, but as soon as we tried to lift them to slip the tape around their bodies in order to measure their girth, all hell broke loose. The sharks erupted into contorting, lashing furies. Their muscular power was extraordinary. Six men couldn't hold one still, as we found out when we called for assistance. But somehow we got approximations of their dimensions and then released them. They reverted at once to their placid mood. The university carpenters would build us a prototype shark box and we would then fit it with the plastic tubing, pump and battery needed for the trucking experiment. While the carpenters worked, Robert and I had two spare days in which to explore Havana and the surrounding countryside.

On my first visit to Cuba I had found it difficult to find a church that was open – even on Sundays. While travelling I enjoy, wherever possible, visiting old churches and going to mass, especially in countries where the church itself is politically oppressed or desperately hanging on by the skin of its teeth. Out of bed most mornings at five o'clock, it's easy for me to get to an early service and be back for breakfast and the day's work. Over the years, while globe-trotting on sick animal business, I've strained to hear the 'Kyrie' in Prague's impressive St Vitus Cathedral while a May Day military parade rumbled and blared outside, been the only person present apart from the priest during a December blizzard in Iceland, and had my hand shaken for some reason by every member of a large Indian congregation at a church in Arabia where the infidel cross is prohibited from being erected on such a building. In Greenland I'd heard a bishop refer to Christ as 'the harp seal of God' – few, if any, of the Inuits present would have ever heard of, let alone seen, a lamb; and in Southern France I'd listened as a clairvoyant nun of the obscure Antoiniste sect had studied a photograph of the animal to diagnose the cause of a whale's illness – incorrectly as it turned out.

In Havana, during that first visit, a friend from a government ministry had asked me what I would like to see in the city – Castro's famous little invasion boat the *Granma*? The Hemingway house? The cigar factory? La Fuerza fortress? 'No – the cathedral, please,' I had replied, and off we had set in the ubiquitous rattly Lada. In the Plaza de Armas we had stopped outside the tall grey-black building built in seventeenth-century Spanish colonial style. 'There it is – the cathedral.'

I had opened the car door, when my companion said, 'Do you want to walk round it?'

'I want to look *in* it – it contains one of the tombs of Columbus, I believe.' It was immediately obvious that I had embarrassed my guide.

'Er . . . I don't think that would be possible,' he explained. 'It is shut . . . for repairs.'

'Okay, let's go to see some of the other old churches then.'

'They may be closed too.'

'All of them? Is religion dead in Cuba?'

'Oh, no – complete freedom of religion, Doctor, it's just that . . . these old places need maintenance, reconstructions.'

'So – there must be *a* church open somewhere. I would like to find one.'

The Cuban looked decidedly uncomfortable. 'The famous Capitol Building?' he offered.

'No, I'd prefer to see a church – on the inside.'

We set off again through the shabby streets of the old city. San Felipe? Closed. Santa Catalina? Closed. 'Is everything being repaired?' I asked.

'Yes, I think so,' came the answer. There were no signs of scaffolding or workmen.

'I don't think there's a single church working in Havana,' I said eventually, as we sat over plates of 'Moors and Christians', black beans and white rice, at midday.

My companion glanced quickly to right and left, and then leaned towards me. 'After lunch we'll try the church of Belem – *I was baptized there*,' he whispered. 'You must understand, Doctor, that I owe my good position in the ministry to my membership of the Party, and it would be . . . *ilogico* . . . to be a Catholic too.' I understood.

That afternoon I struck lucky – the Belem church was indeed open, and I was able to walk around its dusty interior. There were no visitors but us, no clergy or sextons to be seen, no holy water in the stoups, no lighted candles before the side chapels, but there was a microphone on the high altar – the church was still alive. Just. Much relieved at this demonstration of religious freedom, my Cuban friend visibly relaxed as we drove back to the hotel. 'To be frank,' he said, 'I think Fidel and Christ were like two peas in a pod – both *comandantes* of glorious revolutions!'

Subsequently, on my early morning walks in Havana, I discovered another old church, La Merced, that was open though in a sad state of disrepair. I make a point of going to the morning mass, celebrated by a weary-looking Franciscan for a handful of old people whenever I am Cuba. I suppose it's a feeble gesture of solidarity on my part.

Robert and I made the rounds of the few good restaurants in Havana, the Bodeguita del Medio, Papa's and, most famous of all because of its association with Ernest Hemingway in the days before the Revolution, La Floridita, where the daiquiris are so cold they make my chest ache and the Moorish crabs' claws are unsurpassed. Such eating places are always crammed full, but I discovered that a table can be made to appear in the twinkling of an eye by murmuring the words 'guests of the Academy of Science' into the ear of the doorman.

In the West it's only pop stars and 'celebrities' who can perform such conjuring tricks at Le Caprice or L'Escargot, whereas in communist countries scientists, and particularly academicians, are held in comparable esteem. I think it would be rather refreshing if a maitre d' at the Connaught was observed fawning obsequiously before some chap who had just announced that he was, 'The principal scientific officer for pork pig husbandry research at the Min. of Ag., and might Gaston just happen to have free that favourite table in the corner for *dîner à deux*?' and to be heard purring, 'But, of course, sir!'

I was anxious to visit Havana Zoo to see in particular the large breeding group of Cuban crocodiles (the rarest, and reputedly most aggressive, of all living crocodilians) and also the endangered indigenous green, white and pink Cuban parrot. A car from the Academy of Sciences took me there and I was led on a tour by the Director. Half-way round we reached the big cat compound and, as I stood looking at a group of tigers lazing in the sunshine, two keepers appeared, pulling a billy-goat along by its horns. To my astonishment they unlocked the double-gated entrance to the tiger quarters, pushed the goat inside and quickly swung the gates closed again. The billy-goat stood blinking and bemused, while the tigers yawned and regarded him with bored indifference.

'It's feeding time,' said the Director, stating the obvious. At last one tiger got to its feet and walked over to the billy. He moved away a few paces. The tiger padded after him.

I was appalled – physically sickened. Of course I'm accustomed to blood and guts, to animals in pain, to wild creatures doing things their way in the wild. But this was something I had *never* seen before, and I could no more stomach it than I could watch a man being executed.

'You feed live?' I said lamely, my thoughts jumbled.

'Of course, Doctor. Don't you do it in Europe? Fresh food on the hoof. Nothing better – or healthier for the cats. No risk of tainted meat causing infection.' Another tiger stood up and ambled over, sniffing. The billy-goat was getting the message.

He began to bleat loudly. 'They're not very hungry. No pounce for you to watch,' continued the Director. 'We're too good to our cats. They get fed six days a week.'

Maybe it wouldn't have been so bad if one of the tigers had made a quick kill – the slink run, the ambush, the final sprint, the leap, the precise lethal bite to the neck, like I'd seen in India. A perfect predator killing fast and killing to survive. This was utterly different. One of the tigers ran round to the rear of the billy-goat and seized hold of its scrotum; the goat remained standing and the tiger began to pull slowly, lackadaisically.

'This, *compañero*, is a horror!' I at last found myself able to speak. 'Medieval, barbaric, cruel –' I forgot the Spanish words in the heat of the moment and spat out bastard Spanglish. 'I'm off back to the city.'

'But, Doctor, you're a zoo man, no? A *veterinario*? What is the matter? A goat is a goat is a goat. Nothing.'

'*Mierda*! Bullshit!' I stalked off towards the car-park. The best pet I've ever had – but he was more than that – and the most intelligent, was Henry, a white goat who had lived in the market garden of my home in Lancashire so many years before. Henry, who walked to heel, untrained, better than any sheepdog, when Shelagh and I had gone on walks with him, who could unfasten any latch or catch, who 'hoovered' the grass of fallen leaves in autumn (and stole my strawberries), who could recognize the engine noises of cars belonging to his friends – Henry, *a nothing*?

From time to time the question of live-feeding of exotic animals had cropped up, though I had never before come across anyone who did it, and apparently on a regular basis, with creatures as big as goats. There had been allegations that in certain British safari parks, keepers had on occasion let the big cats kill, say, a donkey, which should have been humanely dispatched before being provided to them. But I'd never found any certain proof that such incidents had really taken place.

Small animals – mice, rabbits, guinea-pigs and fowl – are,

for sure, sometimes fed, live, to reptiles in a few zoos; and, perhaps more frequently, by private owners of snakes and large lizards. Organizations like the RSPCA are opposed to this practice. For me the question has always been, is live-feeding humane and ethical? In the wild, the argument goes, predators kill to live, they're efficient and speedy assassins, it's the law of Nature – red in tooth and claw. Many snakes won't eat, and would rather die of starvation, if denied living food. So what's different about zoos? And now, with reference to what I saw in Cuba, what's the difference between a white mouse being given as a python's lunch and a goat serving the same purpose for a tiger?

I think the answer must be that, in the wild, animals, both predators and prey, are free agents. Both roam free, both take their chances – and the prey animals *do* have their chances. When, for example, a lone lion launches an attack on a Thomson's gazelle, in only twenty-nine per cent of cases does it meet with success. Even when two or more lions co-operate, the success rate only rises to fifty-two per cent. In a zoo or safari park, however, a goat has a *zero* per cent chance of surviving. Also, as with the Cuban tigers, the behaviour of captive predators has been modified by human attention. Animals like tigers live in larger communities than they would in the wild, and are accustomed to regular feeding and unused to hunting – their killing technique can lose its edge, become dulled and too drawn-out. The quick kill of the hungry cat can become a protracted game of lingering death.

With snakes the position is rather different. These reptiles don't play at killing games – they either feed or they don't, and their technique is the same, and as speedily accomplished, whether in the Australian bush or a glass-fronted vivarium. Some snakes, king cobras, for instance, will often refuse dead prey; while others will devour a freshly, and humanely, killed mouse or rabbit. The small animals used for live feeding of snakes – rodents and poultry – in general do not show fear and do not know what's going to happen when they are put into a vivarium where a snake lies silently sniffing the air with

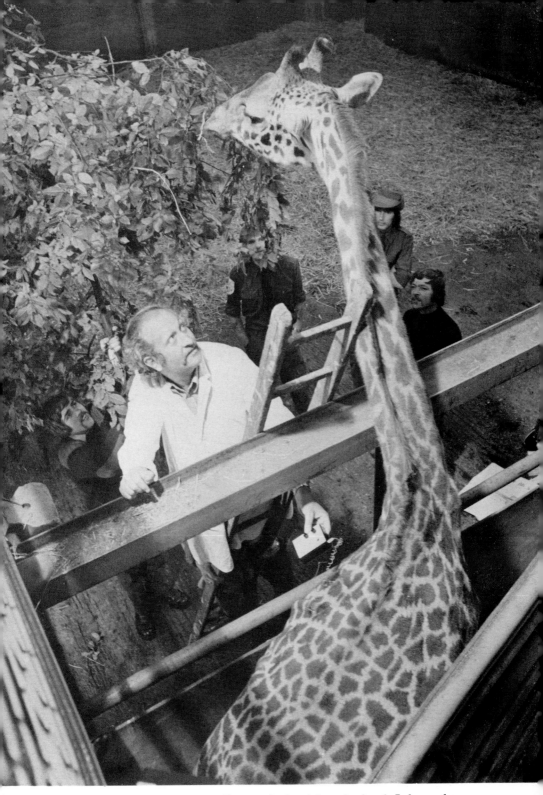

With the acupuncture needles and the 'electric box' I brought back from China. I begin treating a giraffe suffering from chronic polyarthritis. (*White & Reed*)

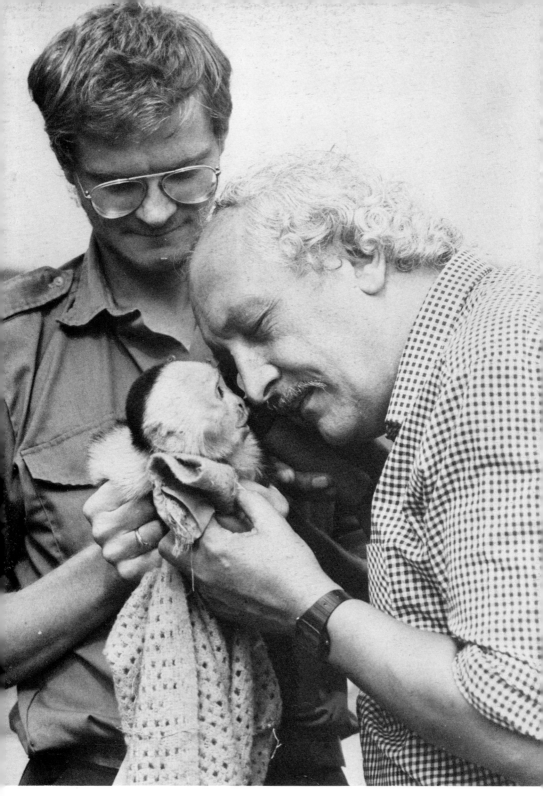

This little Capuchin monkey doesn't know that I delivered him by Caesarian section nine months earlier. (*White & Reed*)

its forked tongue. The end, when it comes, is as swift and humane, often more so, as the way in which they would be dealt with at the hands of a farmer or abattoir worker. Such prey animals again have no choice, no chance; but then, neither do the sheep, cattle and pigs that are slaughtered for people to eat. Snakes deserve to live as much as tigers or naked apes and, unlike the latter, only kill to eat or in defence. They don't overfeed for gastronomic pleasure. In certain circumstances, therefore, for small numbers of individuals and species, live-feeding of reptiles is, I believe, justifiable; but never for tigers and other large predators that are in human care. Good meat, or in some cases versions of the dried or semi-moist complete foods that we give to domestic dogs and cats, is what they should get – always. I went back to my hotel in a black mood, vowing never to return to the Havana Zoo – and I haven't.

Unlike my friend Robert, who had recently had published a collection of his own short stories, which had a distinct, spare, Hemingwayesque style, I've never been a great fan of the macho American writer. But in Cuba, Hemingway is quite a hero, with his house and old haunts on the tourist circuit, and a new marina named after him. Now that my visit to the zoo had been cut short, Robert proposed we should drive out to the fishing village of Cojimar where Hemingway had written *The Old Man and The Sea* and pay a visit to La Terraza, the bar where he used to drink.

It was a heavy humid afternoon as we arrived in Cojimar, an unpicturesque place of paint-flaking bungalows and wooden shanties at the sea's edge. La Terraza was still there, now grubby and fly-blown with a handful of old men sitting at rickety plastic tables, but the long wooden bar and the bar-tenders in white shirts and bow ties standing ready to serve looked more promising. Both of us were thirsty. 'Two cold beers,' said Robert.

'Sorry, no beer,' said a barman.

'Two gin and tonics, then.'

'Very sorry, *compañero*, no gin.'

'Vodka?'

'*Compañero*, I regret it, but we have no vodka today.'

'Whisky?'

'I'm afraid not.'

'Coca-Cola?'

'Alas, no Coke.'

'Make it two tonic waters with plenty of ice, in that case,' I said. The waiter smiled broadly and made a thumbs-up gesture.

'Good ice we have,' he said; then, after a pause, 'but no tonic.'

'I think,' muttered Robert in English, 'we should try a different tack.' Reverting to Spanish, he went on, '*Compañero*, what *do* you have?' The waiter's smile became a joy to behold.

'Rum, *compañero*, and sugar, and I can squeeze the juice of a lime.'

'Nothing else?'

'Water.' He tapped a jug full of grey liquid, so that there was no misunderstanding of the word.

'Well, he's got the wherewithal to make us a daiquiri,' said Robert, on hearing which word the waiter began ceremoniously preparing the drinks with much bravura flourishing of implements and glasses. The daiquiri wasn't at all bad. We sat on the balcony, looking out over the Caribbean, and talked about our ambivalent attitude towards *Death in the Afternoon* and how I'd been to see Hemingway's parrot, which still lived in a bar in Barcelona, and what might bring a man to blow his brains out. As we were ordering refills, a skinny little man with a leathery brown face and wispy moustache came over to us.

'Permit me to introduce myself,' he said, 'Jaime. We don't see many strangers around here these days.' Invited to join us for a drink – he took his rum straight and fast – Jaime went on to tell us of his work as an artist, specializing in the carving of black coral taken from very deep water. It was no tourist scam – he just wanted to talk and drink rum – and indeed we did later go to see his workshop and collection of exquisite coral jewellery. Beautiful as it may be, the taking of black coral – an animal as endangered as the gorilla or black rhino – cannot be justified and it was an embarrassment when he insisted on giving us each coral trinkets to take home. Like many poor people the world over, Cubans such as Jaime are fiercely generous and proud; to refuse such a gift would have been an insult.

During our conversation, accompanied by a steady procession of daiquiris, talk turned to Hemingway and his old skipper, Gregorio. Was he by any chance still alive? Very much so, said Jaime, and still living, with his wife, in the village. Robert was keen to meet the man who, it had often been said, was the original 'Old Man' of the novel; and Jaime volunteered to go to Gregorio's house, not far away, and see if he would like to join us for a drink. 'He's over ninety now, and puts it down to good rum,' said Jaime as he went out of the door.

Gregorio was still a tall man, stooping only slightly, bright-eyed and with an open, kindly face. His lucid Spanish was less drawled and he didn't chop off words in the typical Cuban fashion; this was due, he said, to his having lived in Cuba for a mere eighty years since emigrating from the Canary Islands. As Jaime had claimed Gregorio seemed to benefit from large quantities of good rum; he talked about his life with Hemingway with an articulacy that, even as the day wore on, showed no signs of being influenced by the number of empty bottles of Havana Club steadily accumulating on our table. No, he explained, he was not the original 'Old Man', but he remembered an incident which he thought was the one that gave Hemingway the idea. They'd gone out in the boat from Cojimar and the writer was, as usual, reading on the way to the fishing grounds. Far out from land, they'd come across a small dinghy with an old fellow and a young lad on board. The boy was fishing under the instruction of *el viejo*, the old one, and Hemingway had told Gregorio to steer towards them in order to pass the time of day and give them a crate of cold beer. 'Bugger off!' the old man had shouted when they got near – and so they did. Later, at the end of the day, Hemingway had asked Gregorio to see if he could find the couple again. They had tried and failed, and despite thorough inquiries in Cojimar and the other coastal fishing villages over the months that followed, Hemingway was never able to track down the old man and the young boy.

When at last Robert and I were brimming with daiquiris and Jaime and Gregorio were still happily slugging the fifth bottle of rum, we made our farewells, but not before giving Gregorio a lift back to his home. In the car he told us that he had a large collection of autographs of famous people from all over the world who, mainly before the Revolution, had come to Cuba because of the legendary Hemingway. 'You know,' he said, 'there is one autograph I would love to obtain, one more than any other.'

'Whose is that?' I asked.

'Margaret Thatcher – that gorgeous woman!' he replied.

'You admire our Conservative Prime Minister?'

'What's reactionary capitalism got to do with a hot *chica* like that? I would like to take her to bed!' said the nonagenarian seafarer, who then went on to describe in explicit detail his still vigorous sexual capabilities! I promised Gregorio that, although it was unlikely I could arrange an assignation with the lady in question, I would try to get a signed photograph of her for him. 'To have a picture of Margaret on my wall would put even more lead in my pencil!' he crowed as we finally shook hands.

When I got back to England I wrote to the Prime Minister, describing the old Cuban's devotion (but omitting the more carnal aspects) and before long I received a photograph of her signed 'To Gregorio with very best wishes, Margaret Thatcher'. It is now his prize possession, fixed, as he said it would be, to his bedroom wall.

The university carpenters duly presented us with the shark box. It looked fine and, with the pump and tubes in place, was soon ready for the shark experiment. Professor Guitart acquired the use of a flat-topped truck for a day, and early in the morning we drained the shark tank again in order to grab the biggest of the nurse sharks. As I had expected, lifting it into the box provoked a battle royal. It fought the combined strength of six men, but was eventually settled in position, pinned comfortably with the arched dividers, and provided with just the right amount of bubbling, moving water. The battery was checked and the lid, with its transparent window, was screwed down. So far so good. Shark and box were loaded on to the truck and Robert and I sat on the back of the vehicle with it. The driver would drive around Havana by any route he chose, until he was running out of fuel, then another driver would take over and Dr Fernandez would relieve us.

It promised to be a bumpy, unorthodox way of seeing the city sights. All we had to do was keep an eye on the shark, watch for any sign of it becoming bright pink in the underparts – which might indicate oxygen deficiency, and bang on the roof of the cab if there was an emergency and we wanted to stop. Robert, Anglo-Uruguayan, half Latin, half Anglo-Saxon, is the best conversationalist I know. Acting as nannies to a shark in the warm Caribbean spring, with Robert expanding on the Latin-American world of politics he knows so well, driving through the bustling streets – colourful in spite of the drab buildings – and the traffic with its many American automobiles of the 1940s and 1950s still running, amid the smells of cigars and salt air, would make a pleasant interlude.

And so it turned out to be; off we set from the Aquarium, through Miramar, along the Malecon, up the Avenida del Puerto to O'Reilly – the shark seemed happy enough, although I noticed that, whenever the driver stepped hard on the brakes, the big fish would thrash the unpinned end of its tail left and right. An hour passed, and then another hour. We'd done the Avenida de las Misiones four times and seen the weather-vane in the shape of a woman, 'La Havana', on top of the watchtower of the fortress, eight times, when we turned once again into the wide street that rises up from the sea-wall towards the old Hilton Hotel, the Havana Libre.

We were approaching some traffic lights when they suddenly changed to red. The driver at first braked hard, then thought better of it and put his foot on the accelerator in order to shoot through. In that instant the shark flexed its spine with all its strength. *Boom, boom, boom.* Its tail smashed against the wooden walls of the box. BOOM. *Kerraaaash!* Just as the truck began to pick up speed, the shark box disintegrated. The shark slid back in a gush of water. Lubricated by the liquid, it kept on sliding – right over the tailboard of the truck.

One moment we had a box containing a shark on the back of a truck, the next the truck was continuing on its way with a jumble of wet firewood while the shark lay squirming in the roadway. Without pausing to bang on the driver's cab, Robert and I both reacted by jumping off the truck – determined to be with our animal at all times, I suppose – and hit the tarmac hard, only just managing to keep on our feet. By good fortune no other vehicle was directly behind us. We ran back to the shark – it seemed unharmed, but the gills would quickly dry out in the hot sun. Looking round, I saw to my dismay that the truck, its driver still unaware that all three of his passengers had absconded, was half a kilometre away at the top of the street and preparing to turn out of our sight. In the other direction, two hundred metres away, was the sea-wall and beyond it what we needed more than anything else – sea water.

'Robert – get some water – your shirt, anything!' I yelled. My friend was off like greased lightning while I stood, legs apart, over the shark, waving my arms at approaching cars. A crowd began to gather – there was a babble of voices.

'He's been fishing. Got a biggun. How the devil did he get it up here all by himself? *Dios mio*, did you catch a monster like that from the sea-wall?' A policeman, blue cap and blue uniform, appeared on the scene.

'What's this – a shark! *Hombre!*' He unbuckled his holster

and pulled out his revolver. 'The bastard's still alive, *compañero*, I'd better put a bullet through its head!'

'No, no! It's okay. It's a . . . on its way to the Aquarium!' Thankfully, Robert came panting back at that moment, naked from the waist up and clutching his sopping wet shirt. He knelt and draped the shark's gills with it. 'We need the truck, or some transport, fast!' I said.

'Too big for my motorbike,' said the policeman. 'Anyway, like I said it's alive. I've seen its head move. Wouldn't want that beast biting my arse from the pillion seat.' Everyone laughed, but this was serious.

'A taxi – that's the answer! A tourist taxi!' I exclaimed. 'There's one over there – look!' One of the slightly smarter Cuban taxis that take only hard currency payment for fares was coming up the street. Robert frantically waved it down. A few minutes of animated conversation followed, with the driver talking about 'a danger supplement', and my friend brandishing a fistful of dollar bills, and then it was agreed. With Robert and me at the head end and the policeman and two volunteers from the crowd at the tail, we managed to get the struggling shark into the back of the taxi. Robert sat with it, and I got into the front.

'*Vamos*! Quick as you can. Ten dollars more if you keep your foot down until we reach the Aquarium.'

The shark made it. Back once again in sea water, it swam unconcernedly as if nothing untoward had happened. Professor Guitart's opinion of the toughness of nurse sharks was justified.

I decided to drop the idea of a shark transport box, and look instead at the possibility of using a big, heavy-duty plastic bag containing some sea water and blown up with air or oxygen, as a means of transporting the animals. We knew that it worked with small sharks and other kinds of fish. We tried some experiments with plastic dustbin liners – they were quickly torn by the shark's abrasive skin – and then with plastic body-bags of the kind used for human corpses – they killed the sharks, because toxic chemicals in the plastic leaked into the water. Eventually I had sent over from England some special, thick, plastic bags that are normally used to line certain types of metal beer barrel. These *couldn't* leak poisonous substances, I reasoned, otherwise the brewers, and even more the beer-drinking fraternity, would be up in arms – or flat on their backs. The beer bags worked. They kept the sharks, the water and the air in, and the complete ensemble flew across the Atlantic and arrived without losses or any further trouble in Majorca.

It was all a far cry from the days of my youth in Rochdale, when the only sharks I encountered were the dogfish, true members of the shark family, that we ate straight from the newspaper with a bag of chips liberally doused with salt and vinegar.

7 Arabian Plights

The large, clay-coloured, fat-tailed scorpion lives now in the curator's collection at Chessington Zoo. On reflection, I suppose bringing him back from Arabia in a plastic box at the bottom of The Bag was a double illegality. A potentially lethal weapon in my hand baggage, and no licence to import one of the smaller, but undoubtedly qualifying, beasts that come under the Dangerous Wild Animals Act. Anyway, he travelled well enough, drinking when thirsty from a ball of damp cotton wool I'd given him, and he turned out to be of a species that Lionel Rowe, Chessington's enthusiastic expert on spiders and scorpions, hadn't seen before.

I found the scorpion at sunset on the day I decided that nine years working full time in the Arabian Gulf was enough for my zoo practice. My custom had been each evening when I was in the Emirates to drive up to the top of the Jebel Hafeet mountain range, timing it just right so that I arrived at the summit at six o'clock. At that hour, when the last rays of sun flooded far below across the desert – the ancient sea-bed through which the arid red escarpment on which I stood had been thrust up, lurching askew, by some cataclysmic cracking of the earth's crust – the sky would be a lambent wash of water-colour, flamingo, coral and oyster, and the distant ground, shadowed dunes and seas of pale sand, were stretched out like a medieval sepia print of all the known world. Silence, but for the breeze stroking the rocks. The muezzin's calls for the fourth prayer time of the day were far out of earshot. If I put a tape of Telemann's trumpet music on the Suzuki's casette player, and turned the volume up full, the sound would echo round the peaks as a fitting accompaniment to one of the

most majestic scenes on earth. This magical time lasted for
less than fifteen minutes, and then the indigo dusk swarmed
up from Oman over in the East.

That evening, as I walked across a boulder-strewn ridge, I
stubbed my toe on a stone that glowed like a giant nugget of
Welsh gold. As it rolled aside, the scorpion had been revealed,
at once on the alert, sting arched forwards over its abdomen.
Life in Arabia was getting to be like that – unpleasant surprises, regularly popping up out of a seemingly tranquil land-
scape. Up here in the mountain twilight, nothing was easier
than to walk with old Khayyám 'singing in the wilderness'.
Down there, trying to make some sense of veterinary care for
the wild animal collections of the Emirates, was becoming
impossible. The bedou Arabs who still live a nomadic life in
the deep desert are becoming fewer and fewer. Oil has brought
unimaginable wealth, towns and cities, television and air
conditioning, trans-desert highways and stretched Mercedes
saloons, and the easy, lazy life. The bedou tribesman with
his seasonal migrations, his intricate codes of honour and
hospitality, his hunger and austere diet of camel's milk and
dates with the occasional luxury of locusts or a monitor lizard,
his raidings and feuds, is almost gone, living for us now only
in the writings of Burton, Philby and Thesiger. He has been
changed and corrected – nothing but the husk of his former
self remains. The shadow of his traditions, vain gesturings,
linger, but the substance is vanished.

I had been lucky, through hunting with Sheikh Saeed
bin Tahnoon, to find and spend time with some of the few
remaining truly nomadic bedou. For them, as for their ances-
tors in the burning, barren wastes of the Empty Quarter,
animals and the ways of animals remain at the centre of their
way of life. Sitting drinking warm camel milk from a communal
bowl by firelight, I had learned things that my textbooks on
camel diseases and exotic animal husbandry – even the old
British Army Veterinary Manual which I'd got from my
former partner in Rochdale, Norman Whittle, and which described confidently how 'under fire they are less liable to panic

than other animals', 'in the Sudan at least seven camel breeds are found among the tribes' and 'three stout planks to enable camels to cross ditches were found necessary in the Afghanistan campaign' – things that even such tomes did not encompass.

I had heard from grey-bearded bedou like Mubarak and Ibrahim of the wondrous white camel herds of the Dhafir tribe of Kuwait, of the finest camels of all Arabia, the Batiniya of the Emirates' coastal region. Old Ibrahim had taken me by the hand and walked with me into the desert to show me the *nassi* grass and *'arfaj* bush which he said were better than any food, even the Western food stones (he meant pellets) that he'd been shown when he visited Abu Dhabi, for camels.

'Tell me about sick camels,' I had said to him as we plucked pieces of meat from a goat roasted in my honour.

'If I spoke for the whole of the holy month of Ramadan, I could not tell you all,' he replied. '*Staghfar Allah*, God forbid you should be so unfortunate, my friend, as to see the ailment we call *jarrab*.' He was referring to camel mange – a remarkably severe, and potentially fatal, affliction caused by skin-invading mites similar to, but far more lethal than, dog mange or human scabies. I'd lost a camel once at Belle Vue with just such a disease. 'My son, *jarrab* will kill a camel in the space of two moons. If you see it, rub the camel all over with a mixture of crushed sulphurous rock, red peppers and clarified butter! Beware the *thalath*, a plant of the marshes in the Empty Quarter. It is full of salt and destroys the lungs.' I never found out what this plant, or the disease he referred to, was. 'Sometimes a camel will go lame, but, thanks be to God, it can be healed with the making of a *wasm*.'

'*Wasm?*'

'Let me explain, Doctor. A *wasm* is the burn of a hot iron. Bzzzzzz.' He made a hissing noise.

'A brand.'

'If you say so. Let us imagine you have a white camel which is lame on the right front leg. Then take a dark camel and make a *wasm* on *its* right front leg; *wallah* you will find that the white camel is sound as this stick in two days!' He had struck his camel stick repeatedly against the ground.

'Tell me, Ibrahim, what do you do if a camel has stomach pain – like a man that has taken a young wife who cannot cook and gives him soured goat meat, even though her eyes are like those of a gazelle?' The old man laughed a wheezy laugh through a sparsely toothed mouth.

'Why, then you must make a pudding of barley and milk and dates, and feed it to the camel. All will be well, *inshallah*.' He had poked my knee with a bony finger. 'But tell me, Doctor, do you have good date palms in England?'

'Actually, we don't have any date palms in England.'

The old bedou's face dropped. 'No dates? Then, my friend, you will have many difficulties with your English camels,' he said.

Muburak, Ibrahim's brother, had only one eye – the other had been lost to a viciously clawing, newly caught hawk when he was a boy. He could handle a camel as effortlessly as if it were a labrador dog. To me the camel is a difficult patient at all times – cantankerous, easily offended, prone to discharge its noisome stomach contents all over me at the drop of a hat, a powerful biter – I have seen a man's skull fractured and one eye destroyed by a camel that grasped his head in its jaws – and a kicker of great force and accuracy with any leg. But, while Ibrahim held the camel's head steady, Muburak would take the black *aqal*, cord, from his headcloth, pass it expertly round one of the animal's forelegs, and give a pull. In a trice it was down on its side. Quickly he would bend its knee and throw a loop of the *aqal* about it. The indignantly gurgling camel was effectively immobilized in less time than it takes to tell.

But it was in hawking that bedou such as Muburak and Ibrahim displayed their greatest skills, barbaric though they are in some aspects. I watched Muburak set a trap one day, a trap to catch a falcon. It was ingenious and complex. First he laid out on the ground a fine oblong net set in a framework of thin sticks. Attached to this was a hundred-metre length of

string which, if pulled, would flip the net over to catch anything beneath it. The string led to a hole the bedou had dug
in the ground and in which his son, Mohammed, squatted,
concealed by a layer of dry *nassi* grass. Close to the near end
of the net a pigeon was tied by a short length of string that
linked one of its feet to a wooden peg in the ground. The other
foot was attached to a second string also controlled by the
boy. The third element in the trap was a surprising one: a
tame raven which had a bunch of pigeon feathers tied to one
of its feet. The other foot was fastened to a third two-hundred-
metre-long piece of string which again led to Mohammed in
his hole. Crouched beside Muburak in a hollow edged by
tamarisk shrubs, I had watched through binoculars how the
device achieved its purpose. First the raven was released and
flew high, circling round and round with the pigeon feathers
dangling from its leg. Far away, several miles in all likelihood,
a falcon spotted the black bird apparently carrying a pigeon
in its claws, and came like a javelin to relieve the raven of its
lunch. As soon as the raven caught sight of the hawk, it landed
and was pulled in by Mohammed using string number one.
The boy then jiggled string number two to make the pigeon
flutter, the falcon dived at once to make the kill, and as it
began to pluck at its victim, string number three was jerked
rapidly, bringing the net in its frame swiftly over to trap the
bird. Mubarak ran up and seized hold of the falcon, pressing
its wings close into the body. Out from the hole emerged his
son, who took over the bird, while Muburak produced a needle
and thread from the purse slung round his waist beneath his
dish-dasha. He threaded the needle, passed it through the
falcon's lower right eyelid, over its head and then through the
lower left eyelid. Gently he tightened the thread, forcing both
eyes to close. Deftly making a knot, he bit off the thread and
placed a soft leather *burqa*, a falcon helmet, over the bird's
head, tightening the leather strings that held it in place, again
with his teeth. 'Ha!' he then shouted to me, holding the bird
aloft. 'Look at that! A fine *hurr*, saker falcon – worth thirty
thousand *dirhams*, I swear.'

Bedou like these men were a delight to be with, to sit and listen to their stories of camels, their names and owners remembered even though it might be thirty years before, the ribald jokes about women and young boys, the detailed arguments, with much scraping of camel sticks in the sand to illustrate a point, over tribal and family territories, roots, wells and quicksands, of sandstorms and bad, dry winds and of the good star, Suhail, that is the harbinger of cool weather.

But they were not the bedou among whom my assistants and I had to *work*, however. The bedou-come-to-town, the myriad sheikhs of first, second and third rank and their retinues of latter-day viziers, factotums, major-domos, toadies, courtiers, hangers-on, servants and spies – these were the people we had to contend with in our daily lives, and the intricacies of dealing with them, rather than the relatively straightforward veterinary care of the oryx, cheetahs and gazelles in the zoos and private collections, demanded a Machiavelli more than a Doctor Dolittle.

Before an assistant went out to the Gulf for the first time, I always gave him the same advice. 'Read and digest a copy of Machiavelli's *The Prince*, learn enough southern Arabic, not that you have any hope of understanding bedous in full flow of one of the many dialects, but so that they are not sure *how much* you comprehend of their conversation when you are in their presence. Never lose your temper and, thereby, face, and know that, even in the deep desert at high noon, someone is watching you, nothing is secret.' Chris Furley, our first assistant in the Emirates, proved an exceptionally resourceful survivor under the toughest of circumstances. I have written elsewhere of his acquisition of a Range Rover as a gift from a sheikh, and how the gift was peremptorily taken back when Chris was accused by a gardener of performing sorcery with some blood he had sensibly drawn from a diseased oryx. It was Chris who first set foot in the minefield that was later to endanger all of us – the hospitalizing of sick falcons in the zoo at Al Ain.

No animal, neither camel nor horse, is valued more highly

by the bedou than his hawk. The arts of falconry and the love of possession of these 'kingdom of daylight's dauphins' courses in his blood.

Though other falcons have been brought to Arabia from time to time, the bedou favours only two species which are perhaps best suited for hunting in the desert, the *shahin*, peregrine, and the *hurr*, saker; by contrast, when hawking was at its zenith in medieval Europe, many kinds of falcon were employed, with persons of a particular class or profession traditionally flying certain species. Thus lanner falcons were for earls, merlins for ladies, goshawks for yeomen, sparrowhawks for priests and kestrels for 'knaves and servants'. The large, handsome gyr-falcon of Arctic regions was the king's bird in those days. I have known illicitly taken gyr-falcons, a protected species, arrive in the Emirates as gifts to sheikhs; but, not surprisingly, these hunters of the far north have in general failed to adapt to the blistering heat of the Gulf. The great sheikhs, who sometimes can own a hundred falcons at the beginning of the winter hunting season, do not necessarily treat the noble birds well by modern standards of animal welfare. Within the space of a single season, a few months, they may lose eighty per cent of their hawks, not to disease or injury only, but frequently as the results of the birds returning to the wilderness – to be trapped again, and perhaps even sold back to the original owner.

The sheikhs are the biggest culprits in the worldwide illegal traffic in falcons; they fork out enormous sums for likely-looking birds, ask no questions and pay no more than lip-service to international wildlife protection conventions. Dispensing their oily largess, they have no difficulty in obtaining the hawks they desire from Pakistan or even West Germany. Private jet planes carry their acquisitions across frontiers, politicians and bureaucrats connive in these days when the currying of favour with petroleum-rich sheikhdoms that need to be bolstered against Islamic fundamentalism is the overriding consideration; and greed, as ever, holds sway over all.

Within their kingdoms and emirates they are insulated by age-old feudal systems against the modern world, so many aspects of which they despise with an arrogant and distorted puritanism. Despite their frequent visits to the fleshpots of the West, their love of its consumer hardware, its girls (and, of course, its gold), they are still often suspicious of modern scientific techniques, particularly in medicine, and when it comes to a sick falcon they are slow to give up the old ways of the desert that go back to long before Muhammad fled from Mecca to Medina and initiated the era of Islam.

If a hunting falcon breeds badly, then it must be suffering from *radad* – an affliction brought on by feeding bad meat or because the bird has been cursed by the shadow of an eagle flying above it. The falcon must be taken to an experienced bedou falconer who will burn its face on both sides above the beak with the tip of a lighted cigarette. If this doesn't work, some goat urine and lizard blood will be mixed with the food; and when the animal at last stops eating and becomes thin and apathetic, it is kismet, the overriding will of Allah. *Now* try the European animal doctor and his methods.

In consequence, the majority of falcon patients that we saw in Arabia were chronic, even terminal cases. 'Kismet' was often a dead bird or an inoperable condition that meant the bird would never hunt again and would spend the rest of its days in a dim-lit humid hut. No bedou doubted Allah's decision to snuff out a bird, but he sometimes gave the impression that he didn't think much of the way in which the English doctor had seemingly nudged Allah's elbow. It was a thankless task; in most cases, when treating a sheikh's falcon, we would deal with the bedou falconer in charge of the birds, a person of prestige and much respect in Arab society. We learned early on that such a man would try out all the ancient, often barbaric, remedies before coming to us and *without* telling his master. If we were successful he would display the cured falcon at one of the sheikh's *majlis*, the twice-daily audiences, and describe how he, Abdul or Omar or Hamdan, had laboured night and day with potions made from herbs gathered specially on arduous journeys to some distant oasis, how he kept the bird alive by chewing every morsel of raw pigeon meat for it, and how his brother Faisal or Muhammad or Sharif, had gone up to the *souk* in Dubai, to find some blue stone with which to cauterize the area where the *djinns* that were causing the falcon's depression had housed themselves. He would say nothing of our involvement, however. After the telling of all this in flowery Arabic to the sheikh and a roomful of people, retinue and visitors, the falconer would be given a modest gratuity of a thousand pounds or a gold Rolex watch, and his brother would be put on the payroll.

If the bird died, or the wing would never work properly again, or a foot was a twisted ball of scar tissue when the sheikh called for it to be prepared for a hunting expedition, then the falconer would, at equal length and in just as flowery Arabic relate how, having almost cured the bird, he took it to the English doctor who, it was claimed, had much knowledge of falcon diseases and modern American and European techniques at his command, but *alas*, he had found him wanting, the claims unsubstantiated. This doctor had used the injecting needle, a sure killer if there ever was one, and had given him small capsules which were poisonous. If proof were needed, then he must have bungled things. After all, these infidel Westerners had books and strange instruments, but what did they know about the *shahin* in practice, the ways of the houbara and gazelle, such subtle quarry? Why, he – whose grandfather had flown two *shahin* against an oryx calf in Ibn Saud's hunting grounds – had seen that these English doctors couldn't even follow the flight of hawk and prey in the deep desert when the sky was white-hot, so poor were their eyes in comparison to those of the bedou. And the sheikh had listened and then nodded. He had thought as much.

On one occasion, showing a sheikh by microscope some slides prepared from the lungs of one of his falcons that had died from fungus infection, I had pointed out the fungal spore heads which resembled, after staining by methylene blue dye, pretty fairy trees. I had said, 'You can see the "trees", which are the cause of the trouble, your Highness,' and I had been publicly ridiculed, with considerable loss of face, by the sheikh's falconer, who said that only an idiot might imagine trees growing in birds' lungs – and anyway every bedou falconer knew the cause of the disease was the way the meat was fed or that the falcon had been brought near a woman who was menstruating. Most of the bedou squatting against the walls of the audience room, scratching at the carpet with their camel sticks and awaiting the usual free lunch of roasted lamb and rice, seemed to agree that what I was saying was arrant nonsense.

Based at the zoo in Al Ain, we saw hundreds of falcons every year – a source of invaluable experience for me and my assistants, and particularly enjoyable for Andrew, a keen falconer when he was a schoolboy at Winchester and now a recognized authority on the diseases of hawks and other kinds of bird. Most of the patients came in the cooler months between October and April, and there were two major medical conditions that we had to tackle, the respiratory fungus infection, aspergillosis, that I have just mentioned, and 'bumble-foot', a sort of chronic abscess of the 'sole' of the hawk's foot. Caught early, we could achieve a very high degree of success in the treatment of both conditions; brought to us when the disease was firmly entrenched, we faced serious difficulties.

The bedou particularly liked us to take the birds in for hospitalization; they regarded it in the same way that they might send one of their Mercedes or Chevrolets to a garage for repair, and expected to return and find the bird in perfect running order. Hospitalization was, in principle, something we also recommended for these cases; we could work on them and supervise their nursing at close quarters. But of course, one expects that an owner, told that the bird will be in hospital for, say, two weeks, will come at the end of the fortnight hoping to collect the fully recovered patient. Not in our experience. An owner frequently did not reappear for three or even nine months. When he did, or to confuse matters, when he then sent someone else to collect the bird, it might have been long dead or, if hale and hearty, he couldn't recognize it! The fact that there was a label on the falcon's *wakar al-tair*, the stand on which it perches, bearing its name, was of no interest to him. If he considered that the bird next door, always a better-looking specimen, was *his*, the one he left for treatment, he would lay instant claim to it. There had been some mix-up with the labelling, but, no matter, he was taking *that* bird. Our lay assistants, Arabic-speakers from Egypt, Pakistan, Afghanistan or Palestine, terrified of arousing the wrath of bedou nationals were virtually powerless in such a situation. They are very much third-class citizens in the Emirates, putting up with exploitation and rank discrimination, even though nearly all of them are Muslims, for the sake of salaries that are very high in comparison to what they could possibly dream of earning back home.

We fared little better, neither did the zoo's Director, an old Austrian. 'I'm a UAE national,' they'd say. 'I'm Sheikh so-and-so's falconer or friend. I *know* this is the correct bird. I'll have the police here in a jiffy if there's any trouble. Guess who, under Islamic *sharia* law, will be in the wrong? Finally, if you don't unlock the door to my falcon's room – I'll smash the lock!' Some of them did just that. The birds' rightful owners were not amused when they eventually arrived to collect their property.

Leaving the birds, if they weren't terribly ill, for six months or more with us was essentially a way of having them boarded and treated for free. The drain on the rather meagre drug budget of the zoo was significant, sometimes leading to a situation where we did not have certain drugs needed for other patients for months on end. The owners paid nothing for our work or for the medication and when, at one time, we tried charging them, I got a rap over my knuckles. Sheikhs always get what they want, and even ordinary bedou nationals, wealthy though most of them now are, must not pay a penny, I was told officially.

'But they are not the zoo's responsibility,' I responded.

'They are not included in our contract, which requires us to work solely with the zoo's large animal collection. The number of out-patient falcons is growing to unmanageable proportions. The sick birds arrive at any hour of the day or night – their owners always being given access by the gatekeepers – and they may introduce epidemic disease into the stock.' A separate hawk hospital needed to be set up.

My arguments were ignored and, as for the privately owned falcons not being included in the zoo stock for which we were contracted, I was handed a letter from the ruler of the region which decreed, in Arabic and English, that 'All the falcons in the country and all animals belonging to sheikhs, must be considered as being zoo animals, properly within the purview of the zoo's veterinarians, as they are potential contacts of the zoo's permanent inhabitants.' In other words, the official reasoning ran, they must be treated in the zoo because they might come into the zoo, a tautology that could have been applied equally well to the numerous scavenging dogs of the slums of Zanair, the immigrant workers' township nearby, which regularly raided the zoo at night killing animals such as gazelle and young antelope in their paddocks.

Sheikhs and other well-connected bedou, with a few notable exceptions, had always treated the zoo's staff, particularly the Indian, Pakistani and Afghani keepers (as well as the animals) in, to say the least, a high-handed fashion. No cars allowed in the zoo – so they would drive in for a tour round. Gates closed at six o'clock – they would insist on entrance at seven. If they felt like fun, they would hand lighted cigarettes to the monkeys, encourage their children to throw stones at the ostrich's eggs or at the bears, those despicable animals that everyone knew were just hairy pigs, and so unclean. In 1979 they had stoned a fine old Iranian wild boar to death. Woe betide anyone who remonstrated with such fun-seekers, unless they relished spending a night in jail or, if the sheikh was a high-ranker, being ordered out of the country. If a sheikh wanted a bird to test his falcons on, he would direct the nearest keeper to open its cage and catch it for him – no matter that it might be a bird of paradise or a rare cock of the rock. If he wanted to dump unwanted animals received as gifts – eagles, a leopard or an ostrich – a man would be sent to drop off a box containing the beasts at the zoo gates, normally with little or no notice.

The general attitude of the bedou to the animals in the zoo was strange and often primitive. I remember the President of the UAE, Sheikh Zayed, coming to the zoo and, while driving round, pointing out animals which he considered to be ugly and ought not to be allowed to reproduce – the hornbills, for example. Fortunate indeed is the zoo that *can* breed these fascinating and spectacular birds. He detested mixed groups of animals – gazelle, antelopes and African birds in one immense paddock co-existing as they would in the wild. All species must be kept separate, he ruled, and he came back a year later to check that his orders had been carried out. He wasn't at all pleased when he saw in one enclosure two strikingly different kinds of antelope, a sandy brown and white hornless one, and a black and white one with spiral, twisted horns. 'Why have these animals not been split up as I commanded?' he fumed. 'Do it at once, *now*!' None of the petrified keepers dared tell this Olympian personage that the animals in the paddock were all blackbuck – male and female – and they obediently set about separating the two sexes.

Sheikh Zayed, we found, was a man of unswerving opinions on all things biological. Some kinds of tree were bad and should be uprooted. Some fodder that we gave the animals was 'poisonous' and should be discontinued forthwith. These animals should be sent to his private island, notwithstanding the fact that it was high summer and we warned of the dangers of tranquillizing them in very hot weather. Those animals must be sent from his island to the zoo without delay (on one occasion they numbered ten thousand pheasants) even though the zoo had nowhere to house them. In such a feudal society, the ruler's word is law and truth.

The problem of the hospitalization of falcons in the zoo grew worse. More and more birds occupied cool rooms near our office in the zoo, and two keepers did nothing but feed and water them round the clock. To ensure that only the rightful owner collected a recovered bird, we tried to institute a security system. Everyone bringing a falcon to the zoo would have to sign a chit in the administration building, and we would take a note of his vehicle registration number. Only a man coming with the same vehicle and with the same name as that on the chit would be able to collect a bird. Identification of the birds themselves by tagging or ringing was unacceptable to the bedou; it would be 'dangerous' or 'hinder their hunting abilities' were the usual explanations.

But of course, sheikhs and bedou falconers go by Churchill's dictum that rules are made for the obedience of fools and the guidance of wise men, and they simply didn't co-operate. Chit or no chit, a man would arrive at our office, day or night, and claim a bird; or simply demand to see all the sick falcons. When Chris or I was present it was often possible to send them away by feigning complete inability to understand the language, or disappear by locking the door and hiding in the pharmacy with the lights out if we saw them approaching. I encouraged the growth of dense bushes with judiciously clipped peep-holes in them, outside our office, through which, when sitting at the desk, I could see the kilometre of drive that ran straight to the main gate.

Somehow we coped with the bedou owners who arrived months late to find that their falcons had been claimed and signed for by somebody else. Many of them would take the chit and, because everyone knows everyone else in that tribal society, go to deal with the matter face to face. Others would simply lay claim to another bird as rightfully being theirs, or be prepared to accept the one left behind by the other bedou. Add to that the deep-freeze full of dead falcons that we kept, each labelled, in case an owner wanted to see the corpse of the bird that he'd brought to us in extremis so long ago, and you can understand that the whole business was, to put it mildly, chaotic.

The only part of it that I enjoyed was the surgery, almost

all of which involved 'bumblefoot' operations. While Philip, our Indian lab assistant, held the hooded falcon, I injected liquid anaesthetic into its breast muscle or administered halothane gas through a small face-mask. A couple of minutes later the bird was unconscious. Bumblefoot abscesses, usually caused by a staphylococcus germ that gets into the foot, often because a talon has been allowed to overgrow and prick the sole, are grape-sized lumps, frequently with thick, multi-layered walls like an onion. They may occupy most of the foot where the toes join, and eventually ulcerate; the effect on the bird is chronic pain, difficulty in perching, permanent distortion of the foot and frequently dry gangrene of one or more toes. The vet's aim is to dissect out this gristly ball, avoiding the delicate tendons that control the talons, as well as the nerves and blood vessels. It is almost micro-surgery. My assistants who, unlike me, spent most of the year in Arabia, and dealt with far more cases of bumblefoot, were considerably more skilled than I was at this intricate operation.

After an initial pair of curved scalpel incisions had been made, that came together at each end to form an ellipse enclosing the 'bumblefoot', the tissues were carefully teased apart, keeping close to the outer wall of the abscess capsule. Sometimes it seemed that I was removing all the soft flesh of the foot. Eventually I would be left with a gaping hole, in the depths of which the glistening threads that were the tendons and ligaments so especially essential to a bird of prey lay exposed. After swabbing the wound and dusting it lightly with antibiotic powder, I set about closing up, using silk sutures. Gauze pads as dressings, held in place by strips of elastoplast, completed the operation, and after half an hour I had finished. The falcon was wrapped in a cylinder of blanket cloth to keep it from fluttering its wings and injuring itself, and then placed in a cardboard box in a quiet corner of our office where we could keep an eye on it until it had fully recovered from the anaesthetic.

It was amazing to me that some longstanding bumblefoot

cases, where I felt that I'd almost completely filleted the bird's foot, healed perfectly and hunted again, able to seize houbara, stone curlew or hare in those powerful talons.

It was in spring 1985 that Chris, then our assistant in Al Ain, telephoned early one morning to say that a few days earlier someone had broken the locks of one of the falcon 'hospital wards', and taken what he claimed was his falcon. Now another bedou had arrived, found that his favourite peregrine had gone, and was making a fuss. Typically, falcon-keepers, curator, Director, officials of the Ruler's Department, Uncle Tom Cobbleigh and all, were wringing their hands, sympathizing with Chris's problems, but shuffling off all responsibility for such a crazy situation and offering no help or support. The aggrieved bedou was coming to Chris's office twice a day, delivering threats to take the matter up with Sheikh Zayed himself, unless he got his falcon back or received compensation to the tune of twenty thousand pounds from the English vet. Ominously, he began putting it about that the doctor at the zoo had *sold* his bird!

Knowing how the dice are loaded in such affairs in Arabia, Chris and I discussed contingency plans for a quick flight from the country if it became necessary. It was fortunate that, because he worked for Andrew and me, he was allowed to retain his passport, unlike the direct employees of the Arab government and many companies, whose passports are held by the employer. It was also lucky that he was due to go on leave in a few days' time, and I would be replacing him. 'Keep clear of the bedou,' I told him. 'Spend your time out of the office, working with one of the sheikh's private collections or in distant parts of the zoo until I take over.'

When I arrived in Al Ain, I at once approached the Director with a request that all falcon work in the zoo should cease. He sympathized, but said that the sheikhs wouldn't agree. There was no way of stopping them sending their birds in, and we could not refuse to treat them. Reluctantly, I decided that all treatment of the out-patient falcons would have to be down-graded. All would be attended to using methods that required the bird to be brought back on a daily or weekly basis. None would be admitted for hospitalization. To get over the problem of the diminishing drug stocks in the zoo, I would issue prescriptions – the owners would complain, I knew, but they could do nothing about it so long as I prescribed medicines that weren't kept in the zoo pharmacy. The town of Al Ain is full of chemists who have all the latest pharmaceutical products on their shelves.

Habaish, the owner of the missing falcon, a squat, blue-jowled man with a Hitler moustache and dressed in grey *dish-dasha*, arrived as I expected in the veterinary office on the afternoon of my arrival. By then Chris was already on a Singapore Airlines flight to the Far East. Backed up by two glowering young bedou who typically walked uninvited around the office, picking up instruments to inspect, opening books and going through into the pharmacy to look at the shelves of bottles and the armoury of dart guns and blowpipes, Habaish salaamed me brusquely and sat down in the chair in front of my desk.

'*Wayn* doctor?' he said. 'Where is the doctor?'

'It is I,' I replied. 'I am the doctor.'

'No. *Wayn* Doctor Chrees?'

'Doctor Chris has gone.'

'*Gone!*'

'Yes.'

'Gone where?'

'Out of the country.'

'When does he return?'

'Perhaps never. Can I help?' I pulled a long face, and tried to give the impression that Chris regrettably was gone for good. Habaish frowned.

'So you are the new doctor?'

'Yes,' my emphasis conveying an air of permanence, I thought.

The bedou said no more, but rose, called his friends and they all left.

Chris was on holiday for a month, and whenever Habaish popped in again, at increasingly long intervals, to check that Chris was indeed gone, as he assumed, for good, there I was. He never raised the matter of the missing falcon. Eventually he stopped coming altogether and we never saw him again.

There was never a dull moment working in the Al Ain zoo; apart from the variety of medical and surgical cases in the vast animal collection, the intrigues and Byzantine politics of the all-male microcosm within its boundaries kept me fully occupied. One day I brought some fossils that I'd found on Jebel Hafeet during one of my mountain sunset trips, and showed them to a group of keepers gathered at the gate waiting for the bus to take them home. There were various kinds of ancient mollusc in the lumps of sandstone. 'Look at these sea snails, hundreds of millions of years old,' I said.

They turned them over in their hands. 'Like conches and the oysters I've seen on the beach in Goa,' said one Indian.

'Where did you find them, Doctor? In the creek at Dubai?'

'Oh, no,' I replied, 'up there on the Jebel.'

'On top of the mountain?' an Iranian asked incredulously. 'But there is no water at all up there.'

Like a fool I walked straight into it. 'Not now, there isn't. But millions of years ago there was, when all this desert was at the bottom of the ocean, and animals like these represented the most advanced forms of life on the planet.'

The group of men stood silently looking at the fossils and then the Indian said, 'It is a lie, Doctor. It cannot be so.'

'But that is the way things evolve.'

'Evolution – I have heard that word,' a Pathan from the Afghan border said. 'It is untruth. The Holy Koran cannot be mocked. Allah made things as they are. This evolution is a lie contrived by the godless!'

'Yes, it is so, Doctor,' cried another Afghani. 'Sea creatures were created in the sea. To say they "evolved" on mountain-tops is a heresy, a lie. These things are trickery.'

I put the fossil back in my bag, and kicked myself for

forgetting the anti-Darwinist teaching of Islam. Next day I
was visited by a stern, bearded Imam from the religious police,
who gave me a wigging and warned me against preaching
infidel heresies among the good Muslims in the zoo. 'The
sheikhs are God-fearing men who, by example, demonstrate
the truths of the Holy Koran and they insist that in this
Islamic state their population is not corrupted and lured into
Satan's clutches. Remember, Doctor, that the sheikhs will not
permit ungodly talk.' I remembered how so often, when I
stored my vials of pox vaccine for inoculating falcons in the
refrigerators of the sheikhs' palaces, I had difficulty finding
space between the stacked bottles of vodka and malt whisky.
I remembered the hundreds of spiked receipts I'd been shown
by my friend, the Controller of a certain sheikh's estate (I'd
been there, working with the private antelope collection) for
cash paid out to prostitutes imported from England, Germany
and Austria for stints of two weeks at a fee of £12,000 apiece.
I remembered, and said that I would earnestly bear in mind
everything the Imam had said. 'Good, and God strengthen
you, Doctor,' replied the cleric as he rose to his feet.

There were the men who came offering large amounts of cash
for aphrodisiacs: 'The medicines you must surely give to fortify
the potency of the tigers and gorillas,' they explained. They had
tried eating sharks' meat, a common local remedy for impo-
tence, to no avail. Other visitors wanted dope to make their
camels run faster in the Dubai races. 'Do you not have *something*,
Doctor, that would give my white camel a boost?' one old bedou
said. 'It's legal and above-board here. When I was a lad we
would insert a plug of cannabis into the beast's rectum. That
would do the trick! But now the police catch sellers of cannabis.
We drench the camels with strong black coffee before a race, but
it is not very effective. They say you have wonderful medicine
here for the wild animals, the fleet-footed oryx and the gazelle.
Please give us it so that my white camel goes like the *naf hat*, the
blast of wind off the Arabian Desert.'

There were the Omani gate-men who raised the rumpus on
religious grounds when Chris Furley's fiancée, Karen, came

to visit him, forcing us to find a way of by-passing them through a little-known gate in the boundary fence. After that, when Chris's successor, John Lewis, went to work for us in Al Ain, *his* fiancée, Linden, went out purporting to be his wife. No problem – and it was a delight for me when John and Linden got married a year later on their return to England, and I broke the news in the zoo and was able to witness the confusion writ large on the gate-men's faces.

There were the Egyptian engineer and the Sudani driver who would tap on the door of our bungalow in the middle of the morning and beg a can of beer which they drank furtively, standing in the hallway, and the veiled sheikhas who threw hundred-*dirham* (£20) notes screwed up into pellets at keepers as they were driven round the zoo. There were the keepers, mainly Afghanis and Pakistanis, who came to me for treatment of their wounds, sustained during quarrels which occasionally involved knives; such incidents had to be kept secret, for they were fearful of being deported if the Director or office staff got word of it; and there was the dignified Mohammed Khan, a keeper of hoofed stock who worked alone, far away, at the most distant part of the zoo.

A poor, ever-smiling, infinitely polite man, at the bottom of the zoo's pecking order, he wore a British Army belt round his turban and gave a crisp military salute whenever we drove out to see his animals. One day he asked me if I would do him the honour of coming to his dwelling one evening so that he could provide a meal for me. We fixed a day and I turned up at the hovel made of bits of scrap tin, wood and sacking, as big as a garden hut and clean as a whistle. He was overjoyed that I had kept my promise, and proceeded to brew tea and boil me an egg. He served the egg just as it was on a tin plate and then sat and watched me eat it. It was always slightly embarrassing to dine with Asian friends among the keepers; never did they eat with me, but sat nearby watching, some-times with a group of male friends and relatives, as was their custom. Mohammed Khan's egg was to me as grand and generous a meal as any I've ever had.

There was the gentle Afghani keeper of great apes who told me one day that his brother, fighting with the mujahidin, had been killed by the Soviet army and that he would be gone from the zoo for a week or two. When he returned three weeks later, he reported to me at once, inquiring about the health of his beloved gorillas, orang-outangs and chimps, and informing me that his brother had been avenged; he had killed a Russian trooper. 'I cut his throat, Doctor, as he was climbing out of a blazing tank with his hair on fire. Then I cut off his nose. See.' He took a small canvas bag from out of his baggy trousers, and opened it to show me a wedge of dried brown flesh that had once been a nose.

Always and everywhere there were lies and deceptions. The sheikh who announced, with fanfares of publicity, that he had bred for the first time houbara (or McQueen's bustards) in captivity – he would not countenance the fact that it had already been achieved in Israel (or Occupied Palestine, as he would call it). In fact he'd done nothing of the kind, but had flown in eggs, stolen from the wild in Pakistan, and had them incubated. The gazelles which were knowingly sent with clean bills of health, to join, and subsequently infect, the herd of another sheikh – even though our assistant Peter McKinney had accurately diagnosed them as carrying a serious disease, Malta fever, which can also attack human beings. Typically, by protesting at this irresponsible act and refusing to connive in the cover-up, Peter added to the list of covert enemies we were making. Eventually these grisly chickens came home to roost.

In 1986 and again in 1988 we were humiliated by being informed, out of the blue, that Sheikh Zayed had ordered our resident assistant veterinarian out of the country with immediate effect. In both cases the reason was given as 'the Sheikh's decree'. No explanation, no justification was ever forthcoming or obtainable, despite my most strenuous efforts. Both cases related to the work we had been compelled to do on the islands of the Ruler and his son the Crown Prince. The cause of the edicts was the insistence of ignorant men that

animals *must* be transported, and therefore darted and anaesthetized, in the blistering heat of high Arabian summer. The
lie machines began to operate. When, months after the event,
the Sheikh inquired why there were only six, instead of seven,
sable antelope in his collection, his eager-to-please lackeys
were quick to explain – the English vet, *against* their advice,
had used poisons that killed them.

An Arab friend of mine explained the scenario, using an
actual example. 'You and your assistants don't understand
the Arabic language, you don't know what goes on when you
leave the islands, and you have no way of redressing the
lies and rumours that seep like mist through the Sheikh's
audiences and network of spies, and are just as intangible.
Recently the man who kept a certain sheikh's bees on one
of the islands made enemies among other members of the
household. One night the scoundrels sprayed insecticide into
the hives. The following day the bee-keeper found all the
bees dead for no apparent reason and, horrified, told his
treacherous colleagues. "What a misfortune! But do not tell
the sheikh!" they counselled, shedding crocodile tears. "His
wrath would be unimaginable. *Inshallah*, with any luck, he will
not visit the hives or ask about the bees for many months,
maybe longer, then you can say they died off gradually, from
disease or cold weather." Some weeks later the sheikh did
inquire about the bees, and the bee-keeper's enemies at once
told their master that they had all died and that their death
had been carefully concealed by the luckless bee-keeper. "For
such deceit, see that he is out of the country by sundown,"
ordered the sheikh. That sort of conspiracy is the risk you
run, Doctor, when working on the islands in particular. Not
that *you* would conceal animal deaths, but that *others* would,
and then, when questioned, declare, without your knowledge
– without you ever having seen the animals in question,
perhaps – that you were reckless or neglectful or incompetent,
and then had not reported the loss. Remember that to a bedou
sheikh the word of a bedou camel-skinner or goatherd carries
more weight than that of an infidel Westerner.'

Andrew and I discussed the situation at great length and came to the inevitable decision; working in the Emirates was no longer fun, we would pull out of the Gulf. In September 1988 I made my last journey up to the summit of Jebel Hafeet to watch the darkness well up from the Oman desert. Then I went back down to the zoo and walked round the paddocks of oryx and gazelle and moufflon, the gibbons, hippopotamuses and giraffes. It wasn't pleasant to think that I might never see any of them ever again.

8 Down to the Sea Again

He always swims in hilarious shoals, which upon the broad sea keep tossing themselves to heaven like caps in a Fourth-of-July crowd.

Herman Melville, *Moby Dick*

The broad Comacchio Canal runs into the Adriatic at the mouth of the Gulf of Venice, approximately thirty kilometres north of the city of Ravenna. Its fresh water, or sweet water as the continentals prefer to call it, is neither fresh nor sweet, and bears its share of the pollutants excreted by north Italian civilization down to the dying sea. There are many things in its water that shouldn't be there, but on a January day in 1987 passers-by spotted something that was anything but a pollutant, though it was most definitely not supposed to be bobbing about in the canal on a freezing cold winter's day; it was a baby dolphin.

How does such a creature, barely one and a half metres long, come to be all alone far from the sea? No one knows for sure, but I incline to the view that dolphin infants – this one was about one and a half years old – are like their human counterparts, long in curiosity and short in experience. Just as a child might wander off from its parents to investigate some fascinating item in a world full of magic and mystery, so the dolphin, perhaps wilfully disobeying the clicking under-water messages of its mother and aunts, decided to explore the different-tasting water of the canal mouth and swam in a bit further, intrigued by the grassy banks, the occasional waterfowl, the moored boats and the strange, floating debris. It was all so different from the world frequented by the school of dolphins to which he belonged – the shallow, inshore, salty waters off the estuary of the great River Po. There, though they weren't to know it, the filth in the water nourished the blooming microscopical animals and plants which in turn

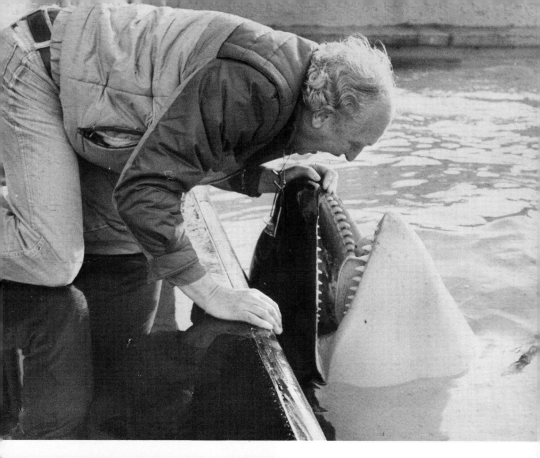

When a killer whale says 'Aah', I have a chance to inspect his formidable array of teeth! (*Brian Duff*)

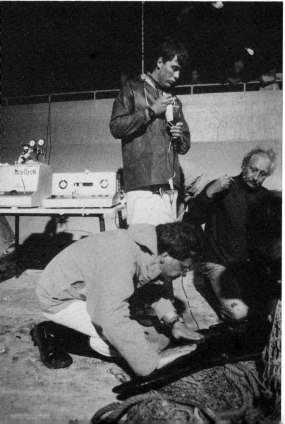

At the Marineland, Côte d'Azure, we washed the blood of a whale suffering from chronic lung abcess.

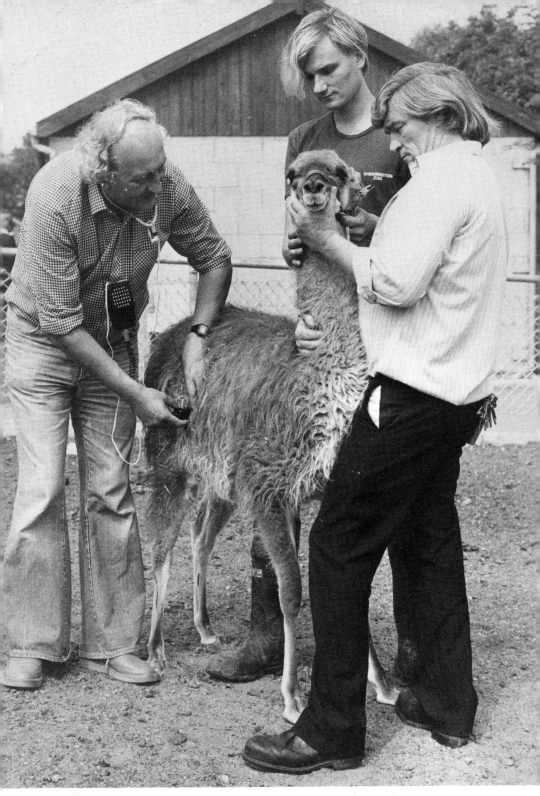

Using the electronic stethoscope to detect the foetal heartbeat in a pregnant llama. (*White & Reed*)

were fed upon by a myriad varieties of tiny, soft slippery things and crusty, jointed-leg, mini-'sea-insects'. Upon this broth dined fish, and the fish attracted the dolphins who, with their sophisticated sonar, could find them in the murkiest water, often little better than diluted sewage, even at dead of night with no moon.

The baby dolphin (who was to become known as Garibaldi after the Italian patriot and soldier and Porto Garibaldi, the place near where he was found) must have panicked when he realized that he was on his own. The excitement of adventure must have turned lemon-sour when he no longer heard the underwater communication noises of the adult dolphins and looked in vain for the familiar streamlined grey shadows of his family as they effortlessly slipped, rolled and dived, soared and banked, in the aquabatic hunt. No joking now! Where was the big bull dolphin who would kill a marauding shark with one belly-blow from his bony beak? Where were the aunts who would take up position, one on his left and one on his right, to escort him when the school was travelling fast away from a storm? Where were his friends, his peers – the other fifty per cent of youngsters who had survived their first year of life in the ocean – the female calf he sometimes chased and nibbled, leaving four shallow love-bite lines on the skin of her dorsal fin, the male that had had a curious lamprey fish attached to him for the past week? I imagine he would have given anything for a taste of salt water, the glimpse of a silver-flashing sardine, the sound of a breaking wave, and the whistle of his mother on whom he still occasionally suckled. But which way to go? Banks, beaches on either side of him. He picked at random one direction in which to swim – it was the wrong one.

As I wrote in *Dragon Doctor*, the Adriatic is a moribund sea; it is expiring slowly from pollution. In 1989 the water's filth fed the explosion of floating algae – blocker of fish gills and defiler of beaches. Who knows what damage this coloured slime inflicts on air-breathing mammals that must surface regularly and find this gunk plastered around their blowholes? Dolphins were already in big trouble in the Adriatic in 1977 when I autopsied a group of twenty animals and found them all to be afflicted by such complaints as kidney stones, breast abscesses, chronic pneumonia and diseased testicles – each disease process related in some way to pollution.

Garibaldi was theoretically in comparatively *less* polluted water while swimming in his canal, but it wasn't salt water. There's a lot of rubbish talked about what happens when cetaceans (whales, dolphins and porpoises) find themselves in fresh water. 'Because of the reduced buoyancy, they have to work harder to rise to the surface to breathe, and soon become fatigued'; 'They die quickly like herring or cod in fresh water' and 'Their skin blisters and falls off'. I've heard it all so many times over the years. In fact, dolphins and whales can survive very happily for many days in fresh water. I remember a white beluga whale from the Arctic swimming way up the Rhine beyond Düsseldorf in the late 1960s. It was there for weeks. In 1969 an old bottle-nosed dolphin spent her last few days of life in the River Severn, but it was a cancer of the roof of the mouth that killed her eventually, not the fresh water. Because dolphins 'drink' efficiently through their skins, I often put a dehydrated dolphin or whale (suffering from, say, diarrhoea or certain kinds of kidney disease) into fresh water for three to four days, so that its body can rapidly and automatically balance its fluid levels. The animals don't tire, don't have difficulty swimming and respond more efficiently than with my original method of introducing a bucket or two of water into them by means of a stomach tube and pump.

It is true that dolphin skin is microscopically different from that of other mammals, and *prolonged* immersion in fresh water will set up changes in its texture. Peeling of the upper layers will occur. Properly managed, with gradual reduction of the salt content in the water, it is possible that a sea-living dolphin's skin could adapt to fresh water and take on the structure of the skin of dolphin species that live naturally in fresh water, animals like the Susu of the River Ganges, the boutu of South American rivers and the 'white flag' dolphin of the Yangtze River system in China.

I discussed this possibility with Professor Sir Richard Harrison, the world-renowned cetacean expert, on one occasion. We agreed it would be an interesting experiment, but an unethical one. One doesn't take unnecessary risks, even for scientific purposes, with our friends the dolphins.

Garibaldi's difficulty in the Comacchio Canal wasn't so much the fresh water, as the absence of suitable food for him and the psychological stress upon an animal so young and isolated from his fellows. Down the coast from Comacchio, at a distance of some eighty kilometres, is the Adriatic Sea World at Riccione, where my friends Leandro Stanzani and Giuseppe Caniglia deftly combine infinite care for the dolphins in their pool with what Hannelore considers to be the most entertaining dolphin show in Europe, and with a real concern for conservation of the world beneath the waves. No mere showmen these, Leandro and Giuseppe put hard cash, effort and ingenuity into scientific work with the threatened dolphins and other marine life of the Italian waters, not least through the organizations they created: the Foundation for the Defence of Marine Mammals and the Study of their Environment, and the Centre of Cetacean Studies, whose conferences attract scientists concerned with marine environmental issues from all over Europe. If anything happens around the coasts of Italy concerning the mammals that live in the sea, the Riccione people are normally among the first to be notified. And so it was with baby Garibaldi.

Leandro at once called his team together, loaded a Transit van with all the necessary gear, and set off at full speed up the autostrada to the north. Just before leaving, he put through a telephone call to me. I was eating my breakfast of Marmite and toast and listening to LBC's half hour of light classical music that goes out each weekday morning at five, when the phone rang.

'I think there's a young bottle-nose dolphin in trouble,' said Leandro. 'Will you be around when I ring later, after assessing the situation?'

Yes, I would be around, I told him, though past experience had taught me that such rescue missions rarely ended successfully. The animal either wasn't where it had been reported and had literally vanished, or it was dead on arrival, or in extremis. Few of the whales, dolphins and porpoises I'd been involved with in rescues after strandings or where animals had gone, like Garibaldi, a-wandering in rivers or harbours, had survived. My autopsies had revealed that many of these sporadic vagrants were diseased – lungs or inner ears full of writhing black worms or brains shattered by haemorrhages provoked by the presence of other flukeworm parasites. Some were unweaned weaklings, others tired geriatric cases come to the end of the road. There had been critical wounds from boat propellers, contamination with oil spillage, and starvation where an individual had been without sea fish for many days and attempts to catch it had lasted as long. But it was always worth pulling out all the stops and *trying*. We'd had our moments of triumph – the pilot whales in Malta, though human error lost them later, a common porpoise at Brighton, some frost-bitten killer whales in Iceland. Some of them, God willing, were still sharing what De Quincey called 'the multitudinous laughter of the sea'.

When the Riccione team arrived at Comacchio they found a small army of men waiting to help them. Police, sub-aquadivers, the Department of Forestry with boats, extra nets, diving gear and vehicles, were all standing by in the freezing mist of an early morning in which the reeds and grasses at the water's edge were encrusted in frost that glistened like diamond dust. There was hardly any breeze, and the surface of the canal water was broken only by the regular rising of the little dolphin for a sharp, short intake of breath. Leandro and Giuseppe saw at once that it was indeed one of the Atlantic bottle-nose species, *Tursiops truncatus*, the 'Flipper' with the permanently smiling curve to its mouth.

With Leandro co-ordinating things on the canal bank and Giuseppe in his wet suit leading the divers, it didn't take long before three nets were set in the water and Garibaldi was gently manoeuvred into an ever-decreasing area where he could be grabbed when he came up to breathe. Having caught dolphins in this manner on many occasions in the past (when for example, I wanted to haul one of the Riccione animals out for a health check), Giuseppe had no difficulty throwing an arm round the youngster's body at just the right spot, immediately in front of the pectoral flippers. The other divers moved in to lend a hand, and a minute later Garibaldi was safely tucked into the padded dolphin stretcher that had been lowered into the water. Carefully, ever so carefully, the animal was lifted into a boat which took it to a jetty where the Transit waited. Before suspending the stretcher in a waterproof framework lined with thick plastic foam, Leandro greased the critical areas of the animal's body (around the blow-hole, the eyelids, and in the 'armpits') with lanolin. Then, without further delay, the van set off for Riccione, Leandro and Giuseppe travelling with Garibaldi in the back and spraying him from time to time with sea water.

The decision to take the baby dolphin to the Adriatic Sea World was the logical and responsible one; it was important to examine him to see what, if any, damage had been done to him by his youthful adventure, and to decide his future with great care. Just dropping him back in the ocean off the beach at Comacchio would have been the easy, but an idiotic, option. If he was ill, if he was not weaned sufficiently to catch and swallow fish – something baby dolphins may not fully master until they are two years of age – if he was alone, marooned as it were, at sea, he would almost certainly not survive in what is an unremittingly hostile environment. I'd seen older, wiser dolphins and whales than Garibaldi simply carried, even towed, several miles out from land by well-meaning animal lovers, only to turn up, beached, dead or dying, somewhere along the nearby coastline within a matter of hours or a few days. But Leandro and Co were determined, if at all possible, to return Garibaldi safely to his own people.

My Italian friend telephoned me from a service station *en*

route for Riccione. 'David, we've got it. A beautiful little thing!' he reported.

'How does it look?' I asked.

'Not bad. A sore tip to its beak where it's been colliding with God knows what. Some skin disease. But it's not emaciated, and it's a strong little *porco mellone!*'

'Get a blood sample as soon as you're back in Riccione. Ask the lab to do a full array of tests.'

'Okay. You'll be coming down, I assume?'

'Of course. In the meanwhile, put him into the separation pool where he can see and talk to your dolphins through the mesh.'

'Do you think it would be best to keep him on his own?' There's always the fear of introducing epidemic disease when a wild dolphin is brought into a marineland. At Riccione we could put him in a portable plastic pool with its own filtration system.

I thought about it for a few moments. Then I said, 'No. Let's house him in the separation pool and put Pelé in with him to look after him.' Pelé is Riccione's brightest and friendliest dolphin. There was a risk of disease transmission, but not a significant one, I gambled, and with modern drugs it's so easy to rid wild dolphins of the parasites which they always carry in stomach, liver and intestines. What Garibaldi needed above all else, I reckoned, was the close contact of his own kind – not just the sight and sounds, but also the touches and caresses. Dolphins are highly *tactile* folk.

As soon as they arrived in Riccione, Leandro took blood from Garibaldi's tail vein and sent it to the hospital we always use down there. Blood analysis is the lynch-pin of cetacean medicine. You'd be surprised what we can learn from a few teaspoonfuls of blood: the sex of an animal (important often with newly caught killer whales); the degree of dehydration in the body; whether a female is pregnant or not (from as early as two weeks after conception); the familial relationships of particular individuals; the required dose of an antibiotic; in the early stages of acute disease, whether a chosen antibiotic is the correct one; the function of major organs, such as liver and kidneys; and the presence of poisons, as well as the routine pinpointing of infections, anaemias, blood parasites, blood cancers and deficiencies of vitamins or minerals. Over a quarter of a century we have built up lists of normal ranges for over sixty blood tests in some of the seventy-six species of cetacean, and my files contain the records of hundreds of whale and dolphin individuals with their 'norms' and idiosyncrasies. No valuable racehorse, no pampered poodle, is studied as deeply and as regularly as our marine mammal patients around the world, a system that improved even further when Andrew and I, together with Professor Robert Turner, an eminent pathologist, set up our own research laboratory in Oxenhope, near Andrew's home in Yorkshire.

Seaside resorts in the middle of winter are peculiarly depressing places, but at least Riccione keeps one good hotel and one first-class seafood restaurant open to help restore the spirits. While hibernation grips the remainder of the town, and the boutiques and beach bars are shuttered, the marineland never sleeps but continues to maintain its animals' health, not least by playing and working with them, by the never-ending monitoring of the water, the meticulous preparation of vast quantities of food imported from the North Sea, the servicing of the pumps, filters and chemical dosers that must withstand the ravages of sea water and chlorine, the training of staff and the organization of study courses. Everyone, both human and dolphin, was excited at the arrival of Garibaldi. When he was lowered into the separation pool where Pelé already waited, and released from his stretcher, the old dolphin nuzzled him and the two immediately swam off, side by side, joyfully leaping from time to time out of the water. Leandro watched as Pelé positioned himself with the tip of his beak or one flipper just under the baby's chest when they dived the first few times, just in case the little dolphin needed any assistance in surfacing to 'blow'. The other dolphins pressed themselves hard up against the mesh to watch what was going on with wide eyes, and the level of communication noises in the pool (chattering a welcome to the newcomer, I suppose) rose dramatically.

I drove down from Bologna in the evening and caught my first glimpse of Garibaldi swimming under the protective wing-like flipper of Pelé in the glow of the pool's floodlights. Leandro was right: he was a beauty. Preferring to make an examination in daylight, I arranged to catch him early the following morning, and Leandro, Giuseppe and I went off to have dinner in *Il Pescatore* with Dr Notarbartolo, an Italian marine biologist. Over mantis shrimps, linguini with pesto sauce and Brunello wine, we discussed Garibaldi's future. All of us were in total agreement that the baby dolphin should go back to the sea. But first he had to be fully fit; and second, we had to find him a family. Sadly, there was no way of helping him to rejoin his biological mother, but we were resolved to provide him with foster parents at least. Unlike some animals (lions, for example) dolphins, with the exception of a very few macho males, are loving and concerned about their own kind, particularly the young, weak and the very old – models of Christian virtue, one might say, and St Francis of Assisi would no doubt have agreed.

'Garibaldi goes when we have done three things,' I repeated, 'made certain he's healthy, satisfied ourselves that he's weaned enough to survive on fish, and found a school of *Tursiops* in the Adriatic, somewhere between here and Venice, ideally in the centre of that zone near Comacchio.' We could begin with the first two objectives the next day. The search for a suitable school of dolphins would depend on what we found out about Garibaldi's physical condition. 'Then, when you're happy that all is well with our *bambino*,' said Notarbartolo, '*I'll* organize an aircraft to go dolphin-spotting.'

Garibaldi wasn't well. The end of his beak was raw and inflamed, he was covered in the tiny black freckles that indicate pox infection, one lung was congested, and, most important of all, his blood analysis revealed evidence of infection. What was more, he showed no interest in solid food in the form of small herring thrown into his pool on that first day. 'Maybe he was still fully on a milk diet,' said Leandro, somewhat gloomily. 'Injections of amoxycillin, and force-feeding of half a kilo of fish twice a day,' was my response. 'He's probably overwhelmed by all the fuss being made of him!'

It was our good fortune that I turned out to be right, or perhaps Garibaldi did not relish a repeat of the painless but undignified experience of having his jaws held open by wet towels, top and bottom, while herring, lubricated with cod liver oil, were slid, head first, by the person with the smallest hand (usually me) over the back of his tongue. In any event we only had to force-feed him twice. The next day he chased and snatched a herring sinking through the water and swallowed it. And then another. Leandro and Giuseppe cracked a bottle of *spumante* when he'd scoffed his half kilo. One of the necessary conditions for his release had been fulfilled, and with him gobbling whole herring, daily injections would no longer be required. The antibiotic and other medicines could be secreted within the gills of a fish, along with a special vitamin tablet.

The baby dolphin did not respond to my treatment as rapidly as I had hoped, and as the days turned into weeks, more blood analyses were needed and several changes in medication. At last, however, Garibaldi's body, which had perhaps had its resistance reduced by pollution, did begin to heal satisfactorily. The numbers on the computer print-outs from the laboratory crept closer to the normal values for Adriatic bottle-nose dolphins. By March we met in conference and decided that the time had come when we could safely begin planning Garibaldi's return to what we intended would definitely *not* be 'the lonely sea and the sky'. My Italian friends had the idea of marking the baby in some way so that he might be recognized, watched out for, by fishermen and marine biologists in the future.

Horses can be branded, cows can be tagged, pigs can have their ears tattooed; it's not quite so easy with dolphins. Tattoos fade from their skins, for their healing powers are much faster than those of other mammals. Metal or plastic tags inserted into the dorsal fin or tail flukes are easily torn out in the boisterous life at sea. Electronic chips under the skin weren't the answer, though they may be the ideal method of the future for identifying all sorts of animals, provided they are at closer quarters. We required something that could be viewed at a distance, perhaps through binoculars, which was more or less of a permanent nature, and which, above all, was humane. The best idea was to freeze-brand Garibaldi with the simple letter G on one side of his dorsal fin. It was agreed that Leandro should arrange for a G-shaped branding iron to be made, and I gave him the formula for a special low-temperature mixture of dry ice and an alcohol.

Classic fire-branding, cowboy-film style, undoubtedly hurts like hell, albeit for a short time; freeze-branding is much kinder, the intense cold instantly numbing the skin nerves. One day we hauled the baby dolphin out of his pool, dried the skin on the left side of his dorsal and pressed the G-brand against it for a few seconds, after cooling the metal instrument by immersion in the dry ice and alcohol mixture. At first the brand didn't seem very distinct, but after some days had passed there was a perfectly white G standing out sharply against the grey of the dolphin. It was easily visible at a hundred metres through binoculars. Now all depended on Dr Notarbartolo and his colleague Dr di Natale finding some dolphins that Garibaldi could join.

Flying out of Rimini airport in a small, single-engine aircraft, Dr di Natale spent many days going up and down the coastal waters searching for dolphin schools of a reasonable size. In bad weather, or even if there was some choppy water, his hunt had to be called off; you can't spot the wave-like grey fins of grey dolphins in grey waves, as I knew only too well from many similar expeditions in the Florida Keys in the late 1960s. On good days however, when the water is clear and glass-calm, an experienced observer can easily count dolphins, estimate their lengths, and even hazard a guess at their sexes, from the air. But the Adriatic in March is frequently storm-lashed, and its water cloudy with stirred-up sand – di Natale and Garibaldi were up against the weather!

And then, on 12 March, they struck lucky. In bright light over an oily, swelling sea, di Natale looked down for the hundredth time that morning and saw what he had been looking for: a school of bottle-nose dolphins about thirty-strong, with at least three calves among them, feeding leisurely at a point some seventeen kilometres east of the port of Rimini. His radio message was relayed by telephone to Leandro at Riccione. '*Ma-donna*! We've found Garibaldi a family!' he yelled. It was 'all hands to the pumps' to get the baby dolphin ready, Giuseppe and two of his lady dolphin-handlers changed into their wet suits and prepared to catch the animal, while Leandro and the others put all the gear into the Transit van and made arrangements for a police escort on the short journey to Rimini. The coastguards volunteered two fast patrol boats, and their crews were already standing by in Rimini port with the engines ticking over.

One hour later, greased all over with lanolin and having been given a final protective long-acting injection of antibiotic, Garibaldi made the second, and I hope final, road journey of his life, accompanied by the wail of a police siren and flashing blue lights. At Rimini he was carried in his stretcher on board one of the patrol boats and, as soon as he was comfortable, the vessel, with its escort, moved out towards the open sea.

Guided by map references supplied over the radio from the spotter plane, the patrol boat reached the area where the dolphins were fishing in a little over an hour. It was a cool, bright morning with a sky the colour of a pigeon's egg, a hazy white sun and calm water. The aircraft circled overhead. Leandro, like all of us feeling a mixture of happiness and regret, began to wipe the excess grease off Garibaldi's body with dry towels. The voice of di Natale crackled over the loudspeaker. '*A sinistra! Cento metre! A sinistra!*' There they were – one hundred metres off the port side – dark sickles breaking the surface, the brief shadow of a curved back streaming with spray. The baby dolphin was lifted in his sling over the side of the boat whose engines had at once been stopped by the skipper. 'Wait till I give the word!' shouted Leandro to the men holding each end of the stretcher poles. He leaned over the gunwales, watching Garibaldi's blow-hole. The thirty-second respiration interval seemed like an hour. Then he breathed: a rapid exhalation and an even more rapid inhalation.

'*Go!*' cried Leandro, and the men released the outermost pole. Turning over as he fell the short distance through the air, the dolphin splashed into the sea, and in the twinkling of an eye righted himself. One upward kick of his tail flukes and, like a grey arrow, he dived from our sight. On the patrol boat's sonar machine, I listened to the underwater clicking of the dolphins and imagined I heard a chorus of welcome.

Not long after, as we chugged slowly in great circles, the dolphins decided they'd had enough fishing and moved off at speed. Somewhere among the dorsal fins that broke the flickering surface from time to time until they were too far away to be distinguished, was 'little G'.

Should you take your summer vacation in somewhere like Cattolica, Rimini or Lido de Jesolo at some point in the next twenty-five years (for that is how long Garibaldi may well live if the pollution doesn't get him), and you're lucky enough to come across a school of dolphins when you're out sailing one fine day, watch out for the letter G – and make a point of letting me know. I just want to know he made it.

9 Animals on the Box

I'd be a dog, a monkey or a bear,
Or anything but that vain animal,
Who is so proud of being rational.
          John Wilmot, Earl of Rochester, *A Satire against Mankind*

'Never work with animals or children' – so runs the well-known theatrical apothegm. Over the past fifteen years I've contrived to work with both many times on television and film, and I know by now that there's a grain of wisdom in the advice.

My first appearance on television was with a lion cub, Simba, in 1965. And sure enough, he caused trouble. Simba had been bitten on the back by his father, one of whose teeth penetrated to the spine, setting up an abscess in the bone, and partially paralysing him. Shelagh and I nursed him back to health at our home in Rochdale, and when he had had his surgical drain tubes removed and was walking normally, almost ready to return to Belle Vue, Yorkshire Television asked me to take him to Leeds to appear in the evening 'Calendar' programme. Fine – no problem. Until Simba relieved himself, and left a neat pile of odorously steaming droppings in the middle of the studio floor during rehearsals!

'Sorry about that,' I said on behalf of the unconcerned young lion, the size of a labrador dog, who had returned to lie quietly at my feet. 'Where is there a shovel or brush? I'll sweep it up.' A knot of people had gathered; they were watching the turd as if it were about to explode at any moment.

'Oooh, you can't do that!' said the floor manager. 'Absolutely *verboten*, sweetie. You'll have the whole studio out.'

I didn't comprehend at first. 'Look, I'm sorry about the smell,' I repeated, 'but animals will be animals. Tell me where a shovel is and I'll have the offending turd out in a jiffy. A puff of air freshener and everything . . .' More people came to join the group gazing at the droppings. There was much quiet talk and shaking of heads.

'Darling, it isn't the lion's *shit* per se that's the problem. It's that *you* can't shift it.'

'Why not?'

'Unions, dear boy, unions. That's what they're arguing about over there.'

'You mean which union is responsible for, has the privilege of, de-lion-crapping a studio?'

'Precisely.'

I walked over to the impromptu union meeting. Simba stayed yawning with boredom beside my chair. The floor manager was, of course, right; it was what I suppose is called a demarcation dispute. The building's cleaners, custodians of all buckets, mops and shovels, wouldn't touch the stuff, but weren't prepared to let anyone else do so; the props department, who move equipment around within the studio, were prepared to move the turd for an extortionately large special payment; and the director, an old school friend of mine, Barry Cockroft, was happy to do it, but all the others were adamant that crap, other than the literary variety, was way outside the province of an NUJ member.

'Er ... I'd be most pleased to shift it,' I interrupted. Everyone glared wordlessly at me, rather as if I'd taken my trousers off in church. Being an outsider I didn't even figure in the Byzantine politics of television studios. I walked back to my chair.

Over the years I was to witness many similar incidents where television unions behaved unscrupulously, motivated by a mixture of greed and bloody-mindedness, holding the companies to ransom and occasionally prejudicing the well-being of animals involved in programme-making. Usually, however, I found that even the most intransigent union members would see that *my* creatures didn't come to any harm, though they had no compunction in switching off all the electricity or walking out of the building if a shoot ran one second overtime without them being guaranteed bonus payments that would have astounded Croesus. By explaining the risks to, say, snakes or pigmy hippopotamuses, if *they* were left without heating, it was possible to make arrangements for power, a light, a heater, whatever, to be provided *just* for the animals. People in general make exceptions for animals; when there was a Transport and General Workers Union strike at Belle Vue, years ago, the union exempted the keeping staff from 'coming out', and during the dock strike I had no difficulty in getting a band of striking dockers to unload half a dozen white rhino arriving by sea for Windsor Safari Park. Having said that, I can also remember the strike of workers in Canada where pickets prevented food supplies getting into a dolphinarium, with the consequence that several dolphins died.

Anyway, back to the now cooling but still noisome lion droppings. Time was slipping by. Ten minutes to 'on air' and no one would permit anyone else to remove the stuff. 'The problem is, darling,' said the floor manager as we waited, 'it's sort of unprecedented, you know, nothing in the rule books. Normally our guests don't shit in the studio!'

Five minutes to 'on air' and the anchor man and the director were beginning to look decidedly edgy. Then it struck me. Those droppings out there were Simba's, and as the lion cub was technically mine, so was his excrement! If I'd dropped my watch on the studio floor I'd have picked it up and no one would have thought anything about it. Leaving Simba again, I made a bee-line for the droppings, pushing my way through the still debating union folk. I bent down, scooped up the cause of all the trouble in both hands and marched towards the studio doors.

'Hey!' yelled someone. 'You can't do that. You're not . . .'

'I've done it, brothers. It's my lion's shit, not YTV's! I'll do what I like with it. Anyway, I'm the only fully paid-up member of D.U.N.G., the Distinguished Union of Night-soil Gatherers, on the premises!' Pushing through the double swing-door I made my way to the Gents, flushed the droppings away and scrubbed my hands. When I returned to the studio, a cleaning lady was finishing mopping residual stains from the floor.

'Oooh – you're a cheeky bugger, but at least it's brought things to a head,' said the floor manager. 'The cleaner got an extra tenner for wiping up after you.' A props man glowered as he saw me sitting down again.

Barry Cockroft came over and whispered in my ear. 'Thanks a million.' Simba, still good as gold, placidly peed a large golden pool on the floor at this point and gave a few yawns, but three minutes later the show went ahead without a hitch.

My second television performance was in 1970 at the BBC in London for a programme called 'Pets and Vets' where I dealt with a variety of exotic animals, including a pet potto that belonged to Val Crisswell, an artist friend of mine from Yorkshire. Pottos are charming little animals that most people have never heard of. They are prosimians – members of a group of man's distant primate relatives that also includes lemurs, lorises and bush-babies – and come from Africa. One of the curious features of the potto is the protective shield formed by prolongations of the neck vertebrae, which become spines that actually project through the skin above the shoulder-blades. When the animal is attacked it buries its head in its hands and displays its shield.

Val's potto made a friendly pet-about-the-house in Pickering, chose a cupboard as its den, and happily hunted caterpillars, beetles and millipedes in the garden. A country lover, it mustn't have thought much of 'The Big Smoke' when Val brought it down to the studios and I interviewed her as the typical owner of an exotic pet. For no reason at all, under the flare of the arc lights, with the cameras rolling and me babbling away about what was it like to have a potto rather than a moggy curled up by the hearth, the potto seized hold of Val's nose with his sharp teeth and wouldn't let go. Blood trickled down, and the potto hung on. A spirited Yorkshire lady, Val wasn't the sort to be fazed even by such an alarming situation. Sounding as if she'd got a very heavy cold, she continued to answer my questions with the lower quarters of the potto cuddled in her arms.

'Id's vedy nice habing a poddo in de coddage,' she continued as if nothing had occurred; 'he's maidly nocdurdal, sleeps during de day.' The blood streamed by now, but still she carried on. 'Lubs fruit, specially plubs, abbles . . .' At last the director called, 'Cut!'

'Great telly, great telly!' he bubbled as he came on to the studio floor. 'It just shows how some of these quaint little furry things are a bit more of a handful than you might expect!' The potto was still clamped on to Val's nose. It took two pairs of hands, hers and mine, to prise the creature's jaws open.

'Are you okay?' I asked lamely as we walked to the first aid room.

'Of course I am, silly,' she said, holding a handkerchief to her nose. 'He was just being a potto, wasn't he? Find me an elastoplast and let's take him to the nearest pub. I could do with a beer.'

In 1975 I was back at ITV presenting animal items on a series called 'Don't Ask Me' along with David Bellamy, Miriam Stoppard and Magnus Pyke, where precise scripting and pre-packaged research was the order of the day; I much prefer doing my own research, and have always subsequently been allowed to do so on natural history programmes both for BBC and ITV. 'Don't Ask Me' wasn't much fun, but at least I discovered the delights of working with tiny animals in front of the camera. I still consider my most interesting presentation was the time when I stood in a large glass box full of flying mosquitoes, holding a tuning fork of the same pitch as the sound produced by a female mosquito in search of a mate. A tap of the fork produced a faint hum which instantly attracted all the male insects in the box, and a few seconds later I found myself holding a tuning fork covered with a thick wriggling layer of amorous would-be suitors.

When we flew in some common octopus from the Mediterranean for this live programme, the poor creatures expired *en route*. Surprisingly, however, they still 'worked' even when dead. We discovered that the pigment cells in octopus skin which, by contraction or expansion, enable the animal to blend with its background – a phenomenon I'd hoped to demonstrate – continues to function normally for many hours after their demise. The viewers never knew that the octopus which adopted a pale and speckled appearance against the sandy bed of one aquarium, and then took on a darkly blotched, almost chequered, design when transferred to another with a chess board lying on the bottom, had given up the ghost at thirty thousand feet somewhere over the English Channel long before the programme went on air. There were other deceptions, such as David Bellamy and his demonstration of ostrich eggs with shells so strong that they can bear the weight of a man; but that's another story.

After 'Don't Ask Me', and with my move to Surrey following the break-up of my marriage to Shelagh, I began to work on 'Animal Magic' from the BBC Natural History Unit in Bristol. Under George Inger, the producer, who was to become a good friend, I had a much freer rein with the items I presented. Johnny Morris, the heart of 'Animal Magic', was fascinating to work with. Immensely kind, utterly professional, always good-humoured, he was, as you might expect, a brilliant conversationalist with wide experience of the world of zoos and a deep love for the countryside, as well as being an accomplished musician and singer and a fierce campaigner for Real Ale.

For 'Animal Magic', among other things I prepared unusual foods that people eat around the world – salted woodlice, worms, ants and locusts for example – and sampled these exotic dishes with Johnny on the programme. On one occasion I presented an item about the rare medicinal leech, placing a couple of the beasts on my hand where they immediately set to, cutting painlessly into my skin with their Y-shaped mouthparts, and gorging themselves on my blood. Talking straight to camera, I was vaguely aware that, as the leeches rapidly filled up with blood, the 'overflow' was running down on to the table at which I sat. Glancing down, I saw a crimson puddle beginning to form around my wrist and I tried to conceal it from the viewers as best I could. However, a fire officer cum first-aid man standing in the wings – there's always one such person on duty when a studio is operating – spotted the haemorrhage and believing, wrongly, that I was in trouble, dashed on to the set and started strapping up my hand with gauze bandage right in front of the live cameras!

The best moment on 'Animal Magic' for me was when I did an outside broadcast from Weston-Super-Mare. It was March, and a large herd of donkeys, owned by a man who supplies most of the 'donkey derbys' in southern England with runners, contained many heavily pregnant females or jennies. I had had the idea of taking the children viewers *into* the wonderful moment of birth – of a baby donkey. George could spare a film crew for one day; all I had to do was find a donkey that would give birth on a particular day.

Donkeys, like all equines, are awkward customers when it comes to predicting the date of parturition. They can almost wilfully, one might imagine, delay and delay the moment – until your back's turned. Zebras are particularly deceptive. They can have bellies like big bass drums for weeks after you first swear that birth is 'imminent'.

I went down to Weston-Super-Mare and inspected the herd, which numbered about sixty animals. From among them I picked out the four most heavily pregnant-*looking* females and gave them a full, hands-on examination. Two were on the brink of foaling, I determined, with markedly slackened ligaments around the pelvis, a relaxing cervix and vulva and lots of colostrum in the mammary glands. Live, correctly positioned foals could be palpated in each jenny through the wall of the rectum, and I heard strong maternal and foal heartbeats through my electronic stethoscope. I arranged for the two mothers-to-be to be taken to comfortable and spacious loose boxes where they were bedded down with deep straw, and then I phoned the BBC to ask for the film crew on the following morning. Next day, when the crew was all assembled and ready, I injected one of the jennies with prostaglandin, a newly available, synthetic version of a naturally occurring hormone that initiates the birth process. Nothing happened for half an hour and then, quite abruptly, the donkey became restless and we witnessed the first contractions. From then on the cameraman had his finger virtually non-stop on the button as labour progressed at a cracking pace. Fifteen minutes after the first contractions a healthy black and white donkey foal plopped on to the straw, quickly followed by the afterbirth. Everything had gone perfectly. Mother and foal were in the best of condition, and we had it all on film.

George Inger produced and directed a 'World About Us' documentary on my work in 1976 when he and a crew followed me on my travels through Britain and parts of Europe. To be the subject of such a programme, doing the actual veterinary work as well as coping with the requirements of both clients and film crew, is extremely exhausting, tripling the workload in my estimation. I had given George permission to film anything that happened, provided no one got in the way; black moments as well as golden ones, if they occurred. In return he gave me something rarely offered by television directors: a veto on anything I didn't like when the film was edited.

It so happened that during the three weeks of filming I was called to an interesting case about which I've written elsewhere, involving cheetahs poisoned by barbiturates at Windsor Safari Park. The worst affected cheetah needed intensive supportive therapy, and while setting up a transfusion drip on the unconscious animal, it suddenly began to develop convulsive seizures. Things looked bad, and at one point I thought that I might lose her. I injected anti-convulsive drugs and circulatory stimulants into the cheetah's leg vein; then sat on straw, waiting to see the response, with my finger on the pulse under the big cat's groin. Gradually I regained control over the situation, and in the end the physical condition of the cheetah stabilized. She would go on to make a full recovery. During the emergency I had forgotten all about the film crew working behind me, but when I relaxed and looked round they were nowhere to be seen. George explained later: 'I thought you were in trouble, so I pulled the lads out.'

'But that's what we set out to film – the real zoo vet's life, the tough times, the emergencies, the failures too,' I replied. 'Anyway, you've given me a veto.' Through being characteristically thoughtful, George had missed some potentially dramatic footage.

It was as a direct consequence of the 'World About Us' programme, which was titled 'Zoo Vet', that I first worked for Television South. David Pick, then a director with the Southampton studios, found himself with a crew, a film to be made – and nothing to make it about, when he was let down at the very last moment by a barge theatre company on whom he had planned to make a documentary. Remembering the BBC production about me which had just been transmitted, he telephoned on the Monday morning to ask whether, by any chance, his team could accompany me for the week if I was not leaving the country. 'No money in the budget for overseas travel,' he explained. As luck would have it, I was planning to travel around Britain from zoos to safari parks to circuses during that time. David and the crew could come along; ninety minutes later they were knocking on my door.

The result of the week's filming was an excellent thirty-minute documentary, and I'd enjoyed every second of working with the TVS people. They were ideal for natural history work – fast, quick to grasp opportunities and undemanding of the animals. Later I appeared in 'Afternoon Club' several times, doing things like 'cooking for your pets', and then began working on the highly popular children's Saturday morning programme, 'No 73', which ran for six series up until 1988. 'No 73' was a delight – not least because it went out live, the best, adrenalin-tingling kind of television.

My particular friend on the show was Andrea Arnold, who

played Dawn. Andrea is a lovely animal-nut, totally free of show-biz pretension. We worked surprisingly well together; she has an outgoing, vivacious, Cockney character, and deep empathy with all living things, and I was, I hope, her genial, professional, foil. The majority of animal items which I presented were with her. Every Saturday morning some new creature would be brought to the house that formed the show's centre-piece. There were elephants, hippos, orang-outangs, reindeer – the whole Ark trooped through as the series rolled on. Many of the animals which I predicted might be tricky – camels, bats, pigs, for example – behaved like angels. The upsets came from unexpected quarters. There was the chimpanzee who hated black men, and who happened to be on the week we also had some coloured basketball players as guests. Whenever one of them came near him he would try to deliver a mighty swipe with a clenched fist. There was the puma, 'guaranteed tame', which charged round the house's lounge as wild as could be, and the emu which couldn't get a grip on the smooth studio floor, and exploded into a cloud of flying feathers every time it tried to walk.

A baby sea lion, 'hand reared, cuddly as a kitten', bit me hard, drawing blood, as soon as the camera swung to Andrea and me sitting ready to talk about it. A lithe wriggle, and it slithered away behind a grandfather clock – invisible. We had four minutes to do on the sea lion, and the camera was picking up nothing but the base of the grandfather clock. 'Well,' I said, forcing a grin and trying to staunch the blood with my other hand, 'there goes Horace, our baby Californian sea lion!'

'Oh, yes!' replied Andrea, as flummoxed as I was. 'Tell me, where do Californian sea lions come from, David?'

'From California, Dawn.' Still I could see from the monitor that the viewers had lots of grandfather clock, but not a scrap of sea lion.

'I suppose Horace is shy, David.'

'Yes, I suppose he is.' 'Help!' I thought. 'Still three and three-quarter minutes to go and we sound like dummies.' To our mutual relief, at that moment Horace relented and poked his front end out from behind the clock. The camera zoomed in. I decided not to go and grab him and risk further embarrassment. Being able to see him at least concentrated our minds on sea lion matters, and we managed to get through the scene sounding a little more knowledgeable about the Horaces of this world. Horace played his part by staying half in vision until we'd finished.

There was the time when I presented an item on lobsters, bought live by the property department from a fishmonger in Whitstable. Several of us were looking forward to having a thermidor for Saturday dinner, but we had reckoned without Andrea. She insisted that a driver took the lobsters from the Maidstone studios back to the sea as soon as the show was over.

Once, when I was demonstrating a selection of live spiders, somebody brushed against a glass bottle containing baby black widows. It fell off the table and smashed, and I actually glimpsed the minute creatures legging it for all they were worth towards the scenery. No chance of finding them in the clutter of a television studio.

'This is a major emergency!' said the floor manager, white as a sheet. 'What shall we do?'

'Don't panic,' I replied, 'remember they're only babies. Bodies the size of pin-heads. Hardly lethal. Get some aerosol cans of insect-killer and spray around the scenery.' Many cans of fly-spray were quickly forthcoming from the stores, and the studio was well and truly fumigated until most of the humans were coughing and spluttering. It wasn't enough. 'The cameramen are asking what will happen if some of the black widows have clambered up inside their machines! The shop stewards are making a fuss!' The floor manager kept looking nervously downwards, and shaking his trouser bottoms. Studios are warm places when the lights are on, but quickly go cold at the end of a show; they're also very dry environments. The chances of the baby spiders surviving the low temperature combined with dehydration seemed slim to me, but . . .

'Shall we close the studio down at once?' asked Janie, the

producer, as she emerged from the control room. 'It'll need a decision from the highest levels.' The place reeked of fly-killer, a chemical equally toxic to spiders, and there were many unusually grim faces as people made for the doors with all haste.

Later in the morning I was summoned to a meeting at the top of the TVS building. Senior management and union representatives were there, along with a man from Rentokil, the pest control firm. It being Saturday morning, several had been called from their beds. I felt I was in the hot seat.

'How many spiders were there?' asked the Chairman.

'Two.'

'How long will they live in the studio?'

'Not very long, I think. They're probably well and truly dead by now.'

'How many people could they *kill* before their venom ran out, *if* they're not dead?'

'Look, it's not like that. This pair are so small I don't believe their mouthparts are anywhere near big enough to bite a human being. Black widow babies take many months to grow into adults, and have to moult several times. Even the bite of the adult, though very painful, is rarely fatal. The black widow has an evil reputation, but it's a shy and retiring creature found all over the United States, and it was responsible for only one death every four years *even before* the modern antidote to its venom was available. There are several much more dangerous species of spider around the world.'

'Can you *guarantee* they're dead, or soon will be?'

'Not one hundred per cent, but ninety-nine per cent – with all the fly spray we've just used.'

'That one per cent of doubt is enough for me,' said someone. 'We'll have to close the studio and arrange for everything – cameras, lights, and special flooring, gantries, scenery, the lot – to be treated by specialists.'

'At a cost, I estimate of £20,000 minimum,' murmured someone else, 'what with the studio out of action for a couple of days.'

When the meeting broke up I walked back to my dressing-room, trying to calculate how much damage the literally hundreds of home-bred black widow babies that Lionel Rowe kept in his room at Chessington Zoo could have caused. Needless to say, perhaps, the black widows of TVS Maidstone were never seen again, nor did anyone working in studio A ever suffer a venomous bite – at least not from a spider!

The show went on. Brock is, I think my favourite British mammal, and I was excited at the prospects of at last working with a tame badger on 'No 73'. My researcher, Harriet, had arranged for the animal to be brought to the studio by its owner who lived somewhere near Bath. One hour before my item was due to go on air we were told by telephone that there had been a most unfortunate incident. The van in which the badger was being transported had developed a hole in its exhaust pipe while on the way to the studios, and the escaping fumes had entered the back of the vehicle, knocking out the badger and a fox that was travelling with it. Both animals were still alive, though seriously affected by the carbon monoxide gas, and the owner had promptly turned round and gone back to Bath to seek veterinary attention.

The badger wouldn't be on the show. I needed an animal to work with. Mike, the props buyer, immediately rang round his contacts, but no one had anything that could arrive in time. 'I'll work with whatever you can get me,' I said. 'A guinea pig, or a budgie.' There was now only half an hour to go, and the show had already begun.

'My son's got a tortoise at home,' said Mike. 'I'll go and get it, but it'll take me twenty-five minutes there and back.'

'Do it,' I urged. 'There'll still be just enough time.' Television studios are well-equipped buildings, but one thing they don't have is the odd animal hanging about in a corner here and there. As the minutes ticked by, I paced up and down the corridor outside the '73' studio, wondering what I could talk about if I had nothing to show the millions of young viewers. Me as Naked Ape? A worm from the lawns outside the building? But it was winter, with hard ground; finding one would take much time. A stuffed parrot from props? Ten minutes to go. No Mike to be seen. Christine, my make-up artist, checked me over.

'I've just seen a dog in reception,' she said.

'A dog?' I jumped out of the chair, so that she inadvertently stuck her powder brush in my eye. 'A dog would do fine!' Leaving her standing, I dashed off towards the reception area, one eye painfully full of powder. Sure enough, sitting at the feet of a large, middle-aged lady on a sofa near the telephonists, was a basset hound.

'Ah, good morning,' I said. 'David Taylor. Vet. Not enough time to explain, but I need an animal, a dog, your dog. Would you, could you? For the children's programme.' The large lady smiled sweetly.

'Well, we're here to meet so-and-so' – she mentioned someone I'd never heard of on another programme. 'But you can borrow Clifford, if you like, so long as I can keep an eye on you both. His manners are impeccable.'

'There'll be a small facility fee.'

'How very nice.'

'Now, he, Clifford is a basset. I'm on in five minutes. Tell me some of the background to the basset breed. Do you show him or breed bassets?'

'My goodness, *do I?* Clifford here is really called Sir Clifford Windfall Mandolin of Waterdown. Won Best of Breed at—'

'Yes, yes. Quite. So bassets were developed as hunting dogs, and their long ears—' The lady suddenly looked as if a cold frog had leapt into her ample *décolletage*.

'Ears? *Ears?* EARS!' It was a perfect impersonation of Lady Bracknell, from Oscar Wilde's *The Importance of Being Earnest*.

'Yes, the long ears.'

'They are not *ears*, my good man, they are leathers!'

'Leathers? Oh, I've never heard the term. But better to say ears for the kids.'

'Ears? *Ears?* You'll make a complete fool of yourself, whatever your name is. These are *leathers*. Everyone, but everyone, knows that bassets have leathers. You couldn't possibly take

Clifford on to a television programme and talk about "ears". And you a vet, you say. *Really*! No, I can't possibly allow you to talk so ignorantly about the breed. What would the basset breeders think? What—'

At that moment, saints be praised, Mike Smith appeared, red-faced and puffing through the swing-doors. 'Got a tortoise, Dave!' he shouted.

Leaving Sir Clifford Windfall Mandolin of Waterdown and his leathers to the tender mercies of his indignant owner, I grabbed the tortoise (no leathers!) from the prop buyer, and ran for the studio. Two minutes to my item and I found my mark on the set. Andrea was already in position and looking anxious.

'No badger?' she whispered. Breathless, I waved the tortoise at her. 'What do you want me to say as openers?' she went on. I had briefed her on badgers at rehearsal the day before.

'Ask me what animal lives the longest,' I said. 'Tortoises are the longest-lived vertebrates – two hundred years or more, some folk believe. That'll serve as a good introduction. Then we'll play it by ear. Ask me questions, and so on and so forth.'

The floor manager began to wave his arms. A red light was illuminated on camera one. We were on air. 'Mornin', David,' said Dawn, at once relaxed and cheerful as ever. 'I've got a question I was going to ask next time I saw you here at 73. What's the oldest living animal?'

'Morning, Dawn,' I answered. 'Well, apart from me (ho-ho-ho) the record breakers for longevity are the tortoise family. And I just happen to have a tortoise here. His name is . . . Clifford!'

Janie said afterwards it was a super item – badgers couldn't have been any better. I wonder if there's an in-word for badgers' small ears. If not, I hereby coin one. Henceforth they shall be known as 'nasturtiums'.

After the first series of '73', I began to play more cameo parts in the chaotic plots of the programme. Theoretically the vet who lived just down the road from No 73, I was also variously in costume as Dracula, a butler, Queen Victoria's rat-catcher and other curious characters – even singing and dancing on occasion. As a result, it was decided that it would be prudent for me to apply to join the actors' union, Equity, to avoid causing problems for TVS. An expert can appear on television to take part in items concerning his own field of work without crossing swords with Equity, but when a zoo vet starts marching about clad in Roman armour for a comedy routine – that's different. Obtaining full membership of Equity was simple; I had years of contracts to prove I'd worked 'in the business', and I paid over a fat cheque as a percentage of my television earnings. There was just one snag. My name. 'It's the policy of Equity for members' names not to be duplicated, and we've already got a David Taylor,' I was told. 'You'll have to change your name.' At last, a chance to stride the boards with a resounding appellation: Theophilus Brandenburg or Clint (Zoovet) Concorde, perhaps, if they weren't already registered members!

'I can't change my name,' I answered. 'Absolutely no way will I do it.'

'Well, what about your middle name? Why not use that?' Which meant I would appear as D. Conrad Taylor. It has a certain ring to it.

'Sounds pretentiously double-barrelled. Won't do it under any circumstances!' My mother would have gone mad. In the end Equity agreed to write to the actor, David Taylor, to ask him if he minded me being made a member. Many weeks elapsed before he replied. So long as I didn't go in for straight acting, he would have no objections. I'm sure there can't be a dry eye in the house when I inform you that, in consequence, the great British public, nay the whole world of theatre, will be denied, in perpetuity, the opportunity of seeing me do my inimitable Richard III. 'Now is the winter of our . . .' Sad!

Andrea and I had proved to be such a successful combination on 'No 73', that it was decided to give us our own series. 'Talking Animal'. We filmed the first run of six programmes in 1984, and the second a year later. Working on a lamentably small budget, we nevertheless made what was a completely new and refreshing sort of animal half-hour for children. And it was an utterly enjoyable business, for the first time blending drama techniques of direction with natural history material. We had our moments.

One of the episodes of 'Talking Animal' was all about elephants, and I was very keen to show a live hyrax, the furry creature about the size of a large guinea pig that is both the elephant's closest living relative and the 'coney' mentioned in the Bible (which wasn't a rabbit, as many people have supposed). There aren't many hyraxes in British zoos, and those that there are tend to be timid, hard-biting individuals, totally unsuitable for handling during filming. Eventually TVS tracked down a pair of reputedly tame, privately owned hyraxes and it was arranged for them to be brought down one afternoon to East Dene in Sussex, where we were making the elephant programme.

Everyone was ready and waiting for the hyraxes to arrive, when we received the news that, for reasons I've never discovered, the two animals had expired before even being boxed for the journey. Over-excitement at the prospect of starring in a television documentary? Anyway there we all were, ready to shoot, with the only hyrax available being a stuffed and rather moth-eaten one mounted on a wooden plinth. Desperate situations call for desperate remedies. Maureen, the make-up artist, set to work at rendering this museum piece as lifelike as possible, dropping glycerine on to the glass eyes to give a bit of sparkle, glueing on horse hairs to replace missing whiskers, and touching up the waxy gums with blusher. Now to get the stuffed hyrax to *do* something!

I suggested to the director that we half buried the creature in an open sack, brimful of grain. With some nylon line tied to its plinth, and running out through a hole in the sack deep below the surface of the grain, we could have a props man jiggle it from a distance so that it might look, we hoped, like a hyrax disporting itself in the surfeit of food. Which is how the hyrax eventually 'worked' while I talked about its biological significance. Unfortunately, when we viewed the film 'rushes' it looked so ridiculous thrutching about, as we say in Lancashire, up to its armpits in corn, that we cut the scene out of the final version.

More bad luck occurred on the same day in a scene where I was going to show that elephants are not in the least afraid of mice – nor vice versa. At Belle Vue Zoo in the old days I had often seen elephants and mice contentedly feeding together from the same pile of cereals in the rodent-ridden Victorian elephant house. For 'Talking Animal' a dozen white mice were hired, and I demonstrated the point by letting a couple run up and down the trunk of dear old Ranee, the gentlest, most lovable elephant in Britain and the star of Gerry Cottle's circus. Ranee purred happily, as she often does. The mice scampered up and down investigating the thick grey 'branch' they found themselves upon. A lovely image for the camera – and then Ranee curled the end of her trunk, delicately lifted up one of the white mice, popped it into her mouth as if it were yet another one of her beloved sugar lumps, and swallowed it! All very embarrassing. That white mouse is the only animal I can remember losing in many years of film and television work.

The hairiest moment in 'Talking Animal' filming occurred at Port Lympne in Kent, when we were making the snake programme. I was with Andrea in John Aspinall's famous 'Whistler Room' and the subject of the afternoon's work was the 'milking' of venomous snakes, in particular two Egyptian cobras. John Fowden of Drayton Manor Zoo, a true snake expert and one of the few people I trust implicitly when handling extremely dangerous reptiles, had brought the two impressive-looking snakes down from his collection. One of them had been 'de-venomed' by surgical operation in the USA and was officially 'safe'. (Although when this animal bit me a year later on 'No 73', John came rushing up after my item had ended and I was sucking my punctured finger, and asked, to my dismay, whether I felt okay. 'Yes – why?' I asked. 'This *is* your de-venomed cobra, isn't it?' 'Oh, definitely,' replied

John, 'but you may feel a little numbness. I think it could be beginning to grow the remnant of its venom gland again!' 'Well,' I thought, 'at least death from a cobra bite is more pleasant than that caused by a viper.' I didn't subsequently go numb, I'm glad to say, but some months later I heard that John had decided to stop working with that particular snake. He trusted it no longer.

The other cobra John brought to Port Lympne looked exactly like the de-venomed one, but had its venom glands intact. It was a fearsome beast. When disturbed it didn't hiss by expelling air from its lung, but literally *roared*. It was as mean-tempered as a spitting cobra and as strong as a king cobra. Because it carried loads of venom, this was the one to use for the 'milking' demonstration.

Milking a snake, an important technique in obtaining venom for the purposes of scientific research, consists of holding the head of the animal firmly with its jaws open, and bringing the two hollow, venom-injecting fangs of the upper jaw into contact with a rubber membrane stretched across the neck of a glass beaker. When the snake feels its fangs stabbed through the membrane, it reacts as if they had penetrated the skin of a prey animal, and squirts venom out of the fangs via an orifice close to the tip. The milky poison trickles down to the bottom of the beaker. Snake venom, a complex chemical mixture, contains substances that have proved invaluable in the treatment of human and animal heart and blood diseases, and it is also essential to the manufacture of antivenins, the specific antidotes to snake bites that are life-savers all over the warmer parts of the world. To milk a snake successfully, you require a firm grip on the snake's head and a steady hand holding the beaker. John's cobra was a formidable milch-cow, able to deliver a heftier kick than any fractious Friesian with a tender udder.

'A real demon,' said John, when I asked him about the cobra and my milking of it on film. 'I'm not sure it's *absolutely* safe for you to handle. It's quick, vicious and sly.'

'Very encouraging,' I replied. 'What do you suggest?'

'It might be better if I milked it – I'll put your jacket on so that the close-ups of the milking are of my hands. Long shots you can do without actually laying hands on the bugger.'

'Okay, but what about the beaker? Andrea was supposed to hold that.'

'She still can. So long as she keeps it still, I'll get the venom into it.'

The director and I talked to Andrea about it. She was happy to hold the beaker, even though her fingers would come within a few centimetres of the lethal fangs. We went ahead and filmed all the long shots with me grabbing the snake with a pair of snake-tongs, and then prepared for the close-ups. John put on my jacket, and when the lighting, sound and camera crews were happy, his assistant opened the bag in which the cobra was coiled. It roared at once. John's hand darted into the bag and emerged with a writhing snake held firmly just behind the head. The business of filming from this angle and that angle began. Half-way through, one of the lights flared out. 'Cut, get that mended,' called the director.

'*Pssssst. Pssssst.*' I turned round. John, still clutching the cobra, was trying to attract my attention. 'Here a minute, David.'

I walked over to him. He lowered his voice to a whisper. Andrea couldn't hear. 'Tell those buggers to get a bloody move on,' he hissed. 'I'm losing my grip on the snake. It's worming its way out of my hand!'

I knew just what he meant. A snake is essentially nothing more than a tube of muscle covered by polished scales, and it isn't as easy as you might think to hold even a small one securely. 'Any minute now it'll be free, or have enough room to strike me. Tell 'em to get cracking, because if I feel it going, I'm going to fling it at the nearest wall as hard as I can to stun it at least, so we have a chance of getting away from it.'

Chilled, I went over immediately to the crew. 'Everybody who is not essential – props, make-up, p.a. – out of the room,' I said quietly. 'The snake looks like escaping any minute. If

John throws it at the wall, drop your gear and run!' The light suddenly came back on.

'We can roll now,' said the director.

'Okay, do it,' I said. 'But if John flings the beast, bugger off like blue lightning!' People had begun scuttling for the door, but the cameraman and sound recordist stayed put.

Fifteen seconds. The fangs punched through the membrane and the venom oozed down into the beaker. 'Got it!' yelled the director. 'Cut. Everybody out!'

John turned on his heels and threw the snake down into the waiting bag. He was sweating big drops – most unusual for him. 'Just in bloody time,' he murmured.

Andrea, calm but perhaps paler than normal, asked if I could find her a glass of wine. 'And a large cognac for me,' added John. 'What were you two whispering about just now?' said Andrea. 'And where's everybody gone?'

10 One by One

The animals went in one by one
There's one more river to cross.

Anonymous song

The year 1987 was a busy one for me, both in veterinary work and in animal filming. I did, *pace* David Taylor, my Thespian namesake, some real acting for the first time, playing (in a drama that went out on New Year's Eve on French television's TF1 channel) the part of Ton-ton, the veterinarian uncle of a small boy who discovers a dolphin washed up on the beach. Filming among the topless girls on the beach at Antibes was fun, delivering dialogue in French was not. For RAI, Italian television, I agreed to let them attach a special camera to the eyepiece of my gastroscope when I examined the inside of the stomach of Chu-Lin, the young panda at Madrid Zoo, when he had a bout of gastritis. The pictures, of surprisingly high quality, were then beamed up from the panda house to a satellite and bounced back down to the studio in Milan. With the nicest little television company in Britain, Border Television, I presented a variety of zoological topics on the children's programme 'Nature Trail', including an investigation of that perennial favourite of mine, the Loch Ness Monster. In one day's filming on and around the Loch we recorded several of the classic phenomena that can explain many 'Nessie' sightings: a dark, deformed log floating in sparkling, choppy water; an upturned boat adrift; a line of ducks flying low; ever-moving patches of glassy calm water across a paler breeze-stirred surface; the running line of hump-like waves produced when the wake of a boat is reflected off the sides of the Loch and meets again in the middle; Highland cattle up to their elbows in mud around the water's edge; and a great crested grebe which, with its long neck, can look vaguely monster-like when sense of scale and distance is lost. There was even a bit of a mirage where a warmer layer of air covered the cold water, bending the light. Though I interviewed for the programme an honest married couple who were adamant they'd recently seen the well-recorded large hump, like the keel of a upturned boat, that suddenly appeared and then abruptly sank out of sight in Urquhart Bay and though I know, and have briefly collaborated with, Doctor Rines, the man who obtained the curious underwater photographs of what Sir Peter Scott thought was a plesiosaur, I am far less convinced than I used to be that there is some undiscovered animal in Loch Ness, and now count it to be an outside possibility. A pity, though.

My major television commitment that year was the third series of 'One by One', the BBC drama based on my first five volumes of autobiography. For the production I was script adviser, technical adviser along with Andrew, and to my delight, a regular 'extra'. It was contrived that I did a Hitchcock-like walk-on in each episode, though the producer insisted I was heavily disguised to avoid causing confusion in the minds of viewers who saw me on children's documentaries. Nevertheless, the lady behind the counter in my local post office always spotted me, no matter that I was bewigged, adorned with a red walrus moustache or even had my back to the camera, in the part of a tourist, waiter or a member of the crowd. For close-ups of surgery, done on ingenious models of diseased organs, it was my or Andrew's hands that did the cutting and staunching of artificial blood. All the rest was the actors – for by this time the principals, Rob Heyland, James Ellis, Sonia Graham and Yolanda Vasquez, had really got under the skin of veterinary work. All were animal-lovers, who had no qualms about handling anything from a spider to an elephant, and they were quick to learn how things had to be done. Rob was first-class at faking injections, using the syringe and needle with its shaft broken off and, having worked for a period at London Zoo's veterinary department as preparation before beginning the first series, he always went about things realistically and with abundant enthusiasm.

The animals loved Jimmy Ellis in particular, and none more so than Lock, an amazing orang-outang the BBC brought over from Hollywood. He it was who had starred with Clint Eastwood in *Every Which Way But Loose*, and I had worked with him before on the first series of 'One by One', as well as on a Terence Stamp film, *Link*, that was made at Shepperton.

Lock was an incredibly talented 'professional' among animal actors, with that air of wisdom about him and the tolerant, placid nature that I find so attractive in orang-outangs. He could do a host of things on the command of his handler, Joe, and the signals were largely visual ones, ideal for film work. When Joe made a particular gesture, Lock would belch, pull faces, stick out his tongue, stand on his head, tap his skull to indicate that he thought you were 'nuts' and much much more, and he learned new tricks very quickly.

In *Link* there was a scene where he had to lift a van by putting his hands under the vehicle's frame on one side, giving a heave and then changing his grip to push it right over. The weight of tilting the heavy van was actually taken by a jack-like device under the chassis, operated by the props men and out of sight of the cameras. Lock only had to *look* as if he was exerting a lot of effort. Joe showed him what was required, and how the vehicle would be tipped by the hidden machinery, and the orang-outang then went ahead and did it perfectly in the first take, with lots of mock effort and suitably melodramatic straining of muscles. The director clapped his hands delightedly while Lock ambled over to sit in the Bath chair in which he was wheeled, like a megastar, to and from the set, and waited for someone to push him back to the purpose-built quarantine area just outside the studio.

In fact, Lock played the part of a malign chimpanzee in the film because no equally talented chimpanzee actor could be found. To make him look passably like a chimp, he wore two large plastic 'chimp' ears on a headband, and had his chestnut-red hair darkened by the make-up department. This sort of theatrical business was Lock's life, and he took it all in his stride. Never once did I see him fiddling with his chimp ears or resenting having make-up brushes whisking around his face. He sat, good as gold, and was far less of a nuisance than many actors who fidget, fuss or play the prima donna in wardrobe and make-up departments.

In Britain the orang-outang had to be kept in government-approved quarantine quarters, supervised by me and my assistants when filming. We were responsible for seeing all doors to the studio were closed whenever he went on stage, for having all his droppings bagged ready for disposal later by ministry 'droppings-disposal' officials, for maintaining the disinfectant footbaths at the entrance to his accommodation, for keeping strangers out, as well as for checking his health each day.

It was different when Lock flew over from Hollywood to Holland with Joe and Dave, another handler, for the filming of 'One By One'. Dutch health regulations were less strict. There was no quarantine requirement and he could go for walks wherever we pleased.

Again, Lock turned in a brilliant performance. He was shown, just once, how to throw tomato soup at Jimmy Ellis (who was playing Paddy Reilly, the character based on my old friend, Matt Kelly, the head keeper at Belle Vue) and he got it right straight away – splat on target! Then he had to wreck an office; normally so well-behaved that butter wouldn't melt in his mouth, he watched as Joe demonstrated how a table could be overturned, files of paper scattered, ink spilled and, most crucial of all, a telephone sent crashing through a window. The handler didn't actually throw the latter instrument but merely picked it up and made as if to do so. Impassively Lock watched with his big brown eyes. He got the point. When the camera started turning he was instantly transformed into a raving lunatic. Tables crashed, flying paper filled the air, ink splattered, and the telephone went through the window pane, exactly where the lens was focused, in a shower of glass. 'Cut!' called the director. Lock instantly reverted to perfect gentleman orang, and shuffled over to hold Jimmy Ellis's hand.

Jimmy and Lock sometimes went for walks together hand in hand, and were driven round the flat countryside sitting side by side in the back seat of a limousine. Pedestrians would stop and stare as the car rode by and the distinguished-looking, large-faced, red-haired *mijnheer* looked out at them and occasionally, yes really, gave a red-hairy wave of the hand in the manner of some royal personage. Jimmy's appeal to Lock may have had its roots in the Irish actor's habit of talking to him earnestly in Gaelic. I *think* it was poetry, but whatever it was, Lock would listen intently, apparently entranced by Jimmy's blarney.

Our film locations in Holland were at the Arnhem Zoo, the Amsterdam Harbour area, and out on the dykes near the pretty cheese-famous town of Gouda. At night the BBC had arranged accommodation for Lock in the great ape house at Artis Zoo, Amsterdam. And that is where things began to go wrong.

Orang-outangs are highly intelligent and social animals, endangered in their wild haunts, but breeding regularly in the family groups of many zoos. I'm not sure that they should be living the solitary unnatural lives of film stars. Such individuals are well fed and pampered, but are they happy? Are they not in essence lonely, as so many famous show-biz folk, imprisoned by the adulation of the public, have claimed to be? At least these human glitterati do have the ability, if they wish, to associate with others of their kind – that's their problem, they are often suffocated by hangers-on and fans. Animals like Lock live monastic lives by comparison. Even though they may be born and reared in captivity, never seeing another orang from the moment they are born (such animals are to be found in the USA though almost never in Great Britain), they are still orang-outangs – 'men of the woods' – not pseudo-humans with orang-outang features, no matter how clever and 'domesticated' they may appear to be. Their rightful *domus* is still the forest world of Indonesia, threatened though it is by the destruction wreaked by man.

Lock's overnight accommodation at Artis was a comfortable room separated by a wall from similar quarters housing a family of orang-outangs: father, mother and youngster. There was no direct connection between the two units, no way Lock could see his fellow creatures, but both rooms had a barred grille in place of a ceiling, and there were armoured glass windows at the front of each through which the human visitors looked. The orangs could, of course, hear and smell one another through their ceiling grilles.

One evening when filming had finished for the day, Joe and Dave took Lock back to the zoo and walked with him, not as before through the side door into the ape house, but through the public entrance. For the first time Lock saw the orang family in the quarters next to his. He was spellbound, rooted to the ground for long minutes in front of their window. Reluctant and scowling, he was coaxed by his handlers down the narrow passageway to the back of his dormitory. Who knows what was going through his mind at that moment? It was perhaps the first time in his life, except for reflections in the mirrors of sets on which he worked, that he'd seen his own kind. There *were* people like him who perhaps knew what it was like to be *him* – there, next door, where the oddly disturbing sounds and odours had come from. In a few seconds Joe would have unlocked the door to his room and he would be inside – alone. Lock saw a metal ladder bolted to the wall. Snatching his hand away from Joe's, he reached for a high rung and pulled himself up in an effortless fluid movement. Another hold above his head, and before his handlers could shout his name, he was on top of his quarters, walking across the horizontal bars of the grille. He went on, expectant, exhilarated, and found himself standing looking down into the room of the orang-outang family.

Joe and Dave were already climbing up the ladder calling him. He didn't hear them. Down below the father orang, an old, bigger male than Lock, looked up and did *not* like what he saw. The male he'd smelled for the past couple of days, the one he'd glimpsed through the glass a few moments before, was now *on his patch*, actually putting a hand through the bars, pointing, beckoning towards *his* mate, *his* offspring. Fully mature orang-outangs may look plump and flabby as Buddhas, and wear tranquil, even seemingly dozy, expressions on their faces, but when they perceive a threat they can move like greased lightning and with frightening power. The father orang attacked, swarming upwards from shelf to rope to ceiling bars. Broad, yellow teeth bared, he was prepared to bite the leg off this impudent intruder. Though the bars separated the two males, arms could easily be slipped between them. If he could grab one of Lock's limbs he could pull it in and inflict horrific damage.

'Lock! Come here, Lock! Here, guy,' shouted Joe, clambering on to the ceiling of Lock's room.

But already a strange battle royal had begun, of snatching hands, of jaws pressed close to the bars. The father briefly caught Lock's ankle, but the younger male broke his grip, leaving rake-marks in his flesh. The two gladiators went at it hammer and tongs, nearly but not quite getting into a clinch, always ultimately frustrated by the thick metal rods. Both males were now in a state of high excitement, and the female and her youngster had climbed up to lend their moral support and make threatening gestures.

Lock was a changed character, his blood swirling with irresistible, previously unimaginable emotions. When Joe got to him and touched his back as he weaved back and forth, eluding the clawing hands and counter-attacking with swift jabs of his own, he was no longer Lock the utterly reliable, jobbing animal actor. Suffused with fury, he turned on Joe and bit him hard and deep in the arm. Now he had *another* adversary – but let them all come! The adrenalin spewed out into his veins.

Badly injured, Joe retreated across the ceiling. Leaving off his main bout for the moment, Lock followed him, intent on doing further damage. The expression on his face was different from anything Joe or Dave had ever seen before, but somehow Dave, standing on the ladder and waving a puny stick, held him off long enough to pull his colleague to safety. The two men ran down the passageway and shut the door behind them. Lock returned to the fray, tormenting his original opponent by swinging up on to a roof joist and dangling down by one arm, just out of reach, awaiting his chance.

While Joe was rushed off to hospital, Dave decided to see if Lock was by now in a more reasonable frame of mind. Opening the door leading to the passageway, by just a crack, he peeped in. Up on the roof joists Lock heard the squeak of the hinges, swung hand over hand along the beams until he could see what was going on and, as soon as he caught sight of Dave's face, came hurtling down to attack. The handler barely had time to pull the door shut and turn the key before mighty fists pounded against the woodwork. Lock was now occupying the service area of the great ape house, and no one could go in without his permission. He returned to his perch again on the joists above the agitated orang family.

I was sitting with Jimmy Ellis in our hotel on the outskirts of the city, preparing to enjoy an evening meal of green herrings and Amstel beer, when the message arrived. Would I go post-haste with my dart-gun to the zoo. Lock had gone berserk. 'Can't be,' said Jimmy. 'Not him. Some mistake for sure. Must be one of the zoo's orangs. He wouldn't hurt a fly!' But when the taxi dropped me at the zoo, and I went to the ape house, there was no doubt about it. Through the glass and beyond the grille I could see Lock in his eyrie, looking decidedly vicious.

'I'll demonstrate his mood,' said Dave. 'Watch what happens when I try to open the door.' He turned the key again and gave a gentle shove. Watching through the windows, I saw Lock respond by dropping down from the rafters, lips snarling. He was clearly ready to repel invaders.

'He's defending his territory. Maybe he thinks he's taken the next door family by conquest,' I murmured.

'Or he's holding them hostage,' said Dave, shutting the door with a bang yet again.

The zoo's curator had arrived, and was looking most unhappy. 'You'll have to get him,' he said.

'Can I gain access to the service area some other way?' I asked. 'From the roof or via the skylight, so that I can dart him through some hole or other?'

'Impossible. The skylight is reinforced glass and doesn't open. No other way in – except the door.'

To dart him I had to enter through the door. It would have to be a clean shot, unobstructed by the roof joists, and at not too great a range, if I was shooting upwards. The gas pistol was designed for close-quarters work. The first dart must do the trick, otherwise he'd retreat back into the roof space and I'd be vulnerable moving deeper into the house; but even then, a perfect intromuscular darting would take three or four minutes to work. Only on the cinema screen do tranquillizing darts have an immediate effect. In real life, no matter how potent the anaesthetic used, you have to wait for the chemical to be picked up by the blood at the injection site and transported to the brain where it exerts its effect. Three minutes is plenty of time for an orang to catch and kill you.

I loaded phencyclidine, the stuff the junkies in the USA call 'angel dust', into a two-cc dart, attached a short, collared needle and fitted the pistol with a new high-pressure carbon dioxide cylinder.

'Right,' I said to Dave, 'when I give the word, open the door wide. I'll go in about three feet. Hopefully, that will provoke him to charge me. It'll be too risky trying for the usual arm or thigh target on an animal moving straight at me. I'll hit him, God willing, in the belly. When I jump back, you slam the door as soon as I'm out.'

'What if he makes it to you and the door *before* you're out?'

'Then we're in the cow-pat!'

'Have you got a gun with you if we have to . . . you know . . .'

'No.'

'We have,' said the curator.

'Okay, bring it,' I said, 'but don't dream of using it unless he gets hold of me.' I detest firearms.

When the curator had fetched a revolver from the zoo's armoury, I nodded to Dave. He turned the lock on the door to the passageway and opened it fast. I stepped over the threshold, not feeling at all like James Bond, with a dart gun held out in front in both hands. Animals normally do the unexpected, but on this occasion Lock did just what I had hoped. He came rushing down from the roof, dropped into the passageway and hurried towards me, arms outstretched, eyes glaring and lips curled back. I pulled the trigger and with a sharp crack the dart flew to hit him close to his navel. Abdominal shots are among my least favourites, but I'd chosen a short needle to be sure I didn't penetrate into the peritoneal cavity. With a screech, Lock came to a momentary halt. I sprang back. Dave slammed to the door, and then with a crash it shook in its frame as the orang-outang smashed into it on the other side with all his force.

'Let's hope that the explosive charge inside the dart wasn't a dud,' I said, sweating profusely. About one in a hundred is.

Four minutes later, with no sign of Lock going back to the roof joists and no noise coming from behind the door, I asked Dave to open it cautiously once more. Covered by the curator with his pistol (I never like being protected in this way; suppose my back-up gets an attack of the jitters, and pulls the trigger and puts a bullet through my back!) I looked inside the passageway. Lock was slumped behind the door, dead to the world. He would be unconscious for half an hour at least.

We carried him to his sleeping-quarters and made him comfortable on a bed of wood-wool.

'What about tomorrow's filming?' said Dave, as I made sure Lock's tongue was safely flopped out of his mouth, and administered an injection of atropine to control excessive salivation.

'Lock won't be doing anything,' I replied. 'He will be, like Elizabeth Taylor often was, indisposed.'

In fact, Lock did only a restricted amount of work from

then on; no more walks with Jimmy, no more rides in the car. The film schedule was drastically re-jigged. The sad truth dawned when I had the opportunity to discuss things with Joe, back from hospital with his arm in a sling.

'When an orang goes wrong, he's wrong for good,' the American said. 'I can see it in his face. Back to the States he goes in two days. But I doubt he'll ever work on film again.'

'Do you mean he'll be retired?'

'I think so.'

'To a zoo? But he wouldn't integrate with an established orang colony.'

'No, that's true.'

'So what then?'

'He'll just not work.'

'You mean – just vegetate?'

Joe didn't answer. I had the distinct impression that Lock was going to move from a sort of busy monasticism to the life of a hermit – alone, off show, unwanted, unusable, though with his basic needs adequately catered for. An actor gone mad. But he wasn't mad. Two days later Lock flew back to Hollywood with his handlers; I've not heard of him since.

When we were working on 'One By One' in Arnhem Zoo, the opportunity occurred to film the actors apparently doing some real veterinary work. No models, no fake blood, no plastic prosthetic wounds and 'diseases'. A young rhino had a sore to be treated and so needed to be darted with a sedative, and a newly-born baby chimp needed checking over, and its mother had to have her vulva stitches, put in after a difficult birth, removed. Rob Heyland, with *my* hands for close-ups as usual, took part in these and other excellent unscheduled scenes. There was, however, a most poignant incident which involved a lion.

We had only just arrived in Arnhem when it was reported that an old male lion had been attacked by a younger rival, and had suffered a serious bite wound of the hind leg. I immediately went to see it, and found it to be one of the worst injuries of its kind: a compound, multiple fracture of the tibia, with the lower part of the leg hanging on by little more than tatters of skin. In the well-equipped veterinary clinic of the zoo, we X-rayed the lion under anaesthetic; it was as I had imagined. There was no chance of repairing the damage, and amputation for such a creature was out of the question. The only course open to us was euthanasia – by giving an overdose of barbiturate intravenously while the lion still slept.

In the circumstances, I decided that the anaesthetized lion and its humane destruction (awful word) could be filmed with Rob looking at the X-rays, inspecting the unconscious animal's wound, and then pretending to give the overdose. The sadder aspects of some of the work I have been called upon to do as a zoo vet were worth portraying honestly, and the animal was not being exploited or having his suffering prolonged. So, while Rob acted the part, I sat on the floor of the clinic, out of camera-shot, injecting the barbiturate solution through a rubber tube that ran up under his operating gown and down the sleeve to his hand which held the shaft of a cannula that I had placed in a foreleg vein. Several members of the crew were emotionally affected by what was a most moving scene. When the episode was eventually transmitted, I wonder if any viewers realized that they were, for once, watching the unfaked death of an animal.

As I said earlier, the majority of actors on 'One By One' were happy to handle the animals and did the job exceedingly well. Only once did we have someone lose his nerve, and I didn't blame him.

We were in Oxfordshire to film a scene where the actor walked a fully-grown tiger on a lead over some golf links and then past the clubhouse. The tiger had been hand reared, and came with a good reputation as an obliging big cat. But a tiger is a very, very impressive beast with long fang teeth and wicked claws and even if, like me, you see, mix with, and talk to tigers every day, a fully-grown male on a dog lead is, to say the least, something to reckon with. If, for example, he does no more than decide to go this way rather than that, you don't argue with a creature so powerful and so quick to tap you on the kneecap with a club-like paw if you demur. If he wants to play by putting his forepaws on your shoulders, you will have to take around a hundred kilos of his weight, and let his rasp-like tongue, which can lick raw meat off buffalo bones, part your hair. If you smell frightened to him – fear changes the odour of sweat – he won't like it, and may take a sample bite out of your buttocks.

So I wasn't surprised when the actor took one look at the tiger he was going to take for 'walkies', and went a palish shade of green. I give him his due – having been assured by the tiger-handler, on his mother's life, that the animal was as soft as a Siamese, and having been shown by the director (a) his contract and (b) the tranquillizing rifle that I would have loaded and cocked at all times (not that that would have saved him if the tiger gave the classic neck bite that means instant death) he said he'd have a go. With trembling hands he took the lead and walked a few paces with the tiger beside him, just for practice. Perhaps the tiger didn't think much of Thespians, or perhaps it didn't feel like a walk over the links on that day; whatever the reasons it looked at him and nipped his hand, inflicting a tiny wound.

That was the end of the actor/tiger relationship. Ashen-faced and wobbly, supported by his wife who had come to watch the filming, the gallant fellow went off to sit down with a large cognac. When he recovered, I suppose he dined out on the incident for a full year. How now to capture the tiger-walkies on film? Producer, director, production manager, cameraman, tiger-handlers, everyone – me included – went into conference. The tiger-handler got the job out of his own mouth. 'Look!' he said. 'That tiger's a big baby. It must have nipped him because he smelled wrong or trod on its toes or jerked its lead. There isn't an ounce of badness in him, I guarantee. Sheer fluke it was. Couldn't happen again.'

'Right,' said the director, 'in that case you are *it*. You do the walkies. Put on the actor's costume, and we'll slip in close-ups of the actor's face later.'

Thirty minutes later the tiger-handler, a circus man born and bred, came out of the wardrobe van dressed and ready to double for the actor. He grinned broadly as he collected the tiger from its travelling cage. 'Come on, boy,' he said. 'Let's show these telefolk what a cuddle-pot you are.' The two of them walked a few metres, and then – yes, you guessed it – the tiger turned its head towards him and snapped. This time it was the groin.

When I examined the wound at the top of his inner thigh, moments later, after he'd peeled off blood-stained trousers, it was plain that he'd been within a whisker of losing one, if not both, testicles. There was the second ashen face that morning!

'David,' said the director, 'do you think *you* could do this scene somehow?'

'Not *** likely!' I replied with feeling. The golf links scene was written out.

Filming with the giant pandas in Madrid for the third series of 'One By One' was delightful in many ways. I played the part of a tourist in a café in the Plaza Mayor, and consumed large quantities of gin and tonic, pepper-stuffed olives and serrano ham while sitting where I was told to sit during innumerable takes of a particular scene on a golden sun-lit evening in August. The BBC afterwards agreed to pay only for the tonic water. We stayed for a night in the most charming *parador*, at Chinchon, close to that village's picturesque circular plaza cum bull-ring, and we shot some scenes, with special permission, inside one of King Juan Carlos's palaces. But the best thing, the principal reason for bringing the entire crew to the city, was the re-enactment of the artificial insemination, done three years before, of Shao-Shao, the female giant panda, and the subsequent birth of Chu-Lin, the West's first test-tube panda baby.

To do this meant co-ordinating the filming with a 'real' medical examination, under anaesthetic, of one of the pandas.

It was all arranged for the day when I would be performing various minor procedures on Chang-Chang, the old male: de-scaling his teeth by ultra-sound, taking blood for routine analysis, and inspecting by ophthalmoscope the corneal degeneration of his eyes which I've mentioned earlier. So Chang-Chang would have to play the part of Shao-Shao, Chu-Lin's mother. Luckily, one adult panda looks much like another, male or female. There was the problem, in this instance, that we would be focusing on the rear end of the animal, where Rob would be 'artificially inseminating' Shao-Shao. Nestling within the off-white fur in those parts were Chang-Chang's two large testicles! But by then we were good at faking, although Joyce Dean, the head of the make-up team, was initially dumbfounded when I proposed that she might make a 'scrotum wig'!

My main concern was that filming should not interfere in any way with the work I had to do on the panda, who would be under only a light, short-acting anaesthetic. I explained my strategy at a meeting with the director and principal actors: 'Chang-Chang will be "knocked out" for approximately twenty minutes. There is no way that I will agree to extend that period purely for filming. I need fifteen of the twenty minutes to take blood, scale teeth, and so forth. That leaves you five minutes – to do everything. Then, whatever stage you may be at, he goes back to his sleeping-quarters on his stretcher. There will be no chance of rehearsals with the animal, and so I suggest you rehearse exhaustively with a bale of straw taking the place of Chang-Chang in the operating room. Finally, there will not be enough space around the operating table for all the crew; only the camera team, one sound man and the two essential actors, Rob and Yolanda, can be in there. Lights must be set up beforehand by the lighting men, who should then clear out. The director must peep through a window. Make-up, wardrobe, props and the rest are to stay outside the panda complex. *And* there must be silence. I don't want the animals stressed by the usual brouhaha.'

'How, if we can't rehearse with the animal, can we fit our lines into the action?' asked Rob. 'How do we practise the insemination?'

'Easy. You will rehearse on the straw bale, and inseminate that! And you should have no pre-set lines of dialogue. I shall go over the procedure with you and Yolanda in great detail until you really know all about it. Then you will be in a position to fake-do it on the animal in the five minutes you've got, thinking yourselves into the parts. Say whatever comes naturally. *Be* the zoo vets. If, for example, he defecates while you're working, treat it as I would. Don't laugh and look to see if the director has noticed and is cutting the filming. Deal with the droppings as I would have to, mention it, or not, as you feel appropriate. Clear it away with some swabs or a surgical towel – and carry on. Remember you're up against a time limit that I shan't extend, even if the director goes down on his hands and knees before me.'

'An obvious question, David. As Chang-Chang is male, how do we pretend to put a tube inside his vagina?'

'By not using close-ups, and by passing the tube, masked by your other hand, under his thigh and along the top of the table. The tube itself is thin, transparent plastic – no one will spot the deception.'

For half a day before the filming with Chang-Chang, Yolanda Vasquez and Rob Heyland, playing in real life Liliana Monsalve, one of the Madrid Zoo vets, and myself, worked with the bale of straw. I watched and listened as they practised coping with all eventualities and invented their own dialogue for this key scene in the drama.

I was somewhat nervous when it came to the actual filming, but in the event all went magnificently well. As soon as I'd finished my work on the panda, I looked at my watch and said, 'Okay – five minutes from now,' and the actors took up their positions over the unconscious animal. If I hadn't known what was going on I would have been utterly convinced that Rob and Yolanda were indeed experts, calmly and confidently hoping to make Chang-Chang (Shao-Shao!) pregnant. Six minutes later the old male was back in his quarters, beginning gently to rouse and totally unaware of the strange cinematic sex-change he'd just undergone.

The finished film of the operation turned out to be a great success and by adding on, in a later scene, some real video footage taken during the birth of the baby panda at Madrid, the story of how Chu-Lin, the famous test-tube panda of Spain, came into this world was accurately portrayed.

11 A Whale of a Time

When I'm playful, I use the meridians of longitude and
parallels of latitude for a seine, and drag the Atlantic Ocean for
whales.

Mark Twain, *Life on the Mississippi*

Freya or Freyja is the Venus of Scandinavian mythology. The
goddess of love, and the wife of Odin, she rode in a chariot
drawn by cats. She is also a mature killer whale, caught off
Iceland, and living for the past several years in the Marineland
Côte d'Azur, outside Antibes, Provence.

Soon after her arrival in France, John Kershaw, the English
head trainer at Marineland, trained her to swim to the side
of the large pool in which she lived with two other whales,
Betty and Kim, to roll on her back and present the under
surface of her broad tail-flukes. In that position it was then
easy to insert a fine needle into one of the large tail veins and
draw off a quantity of blood into special vacuum tubes. By
sampling the whales in this manner every month, and having
the blood analysed, we built up a picture of their underlying
state of health. When disease strikes, the blood (particularly
in whales and dolphins, but also in man and other mammals)
is the first to show signs. It displays alterations sometimes
weeks or months before clinical, naked-eye symptoms appear.

In 1986, at one of the routine samplings, I observed the
first shift in some of the white corpuscles that circulate in the
whale's blood. It wasn't much, but it alerted me. I asked John
to take blood again three days later. Two successive samples
are worth ten times more than one; they enable you to detect
trends. The second sample confirmed my fears: there was a
spot of infection beginning to grumble somewhere in the
animal's body. Nevertheless, anybody watching her scoffing
her fifty kilograms of prime fish each day, or racing round the
pool playing with her friends and jumping dramatically during

the shows, would have thought that there was nothing amiss.

Up until that time we had calculated the dosage of drugs such as antibiotics for these gigantic animals by rule-of-thumb guesswork, multiplying the amount known to be needed for, say, a cart horse by a factor of three and then knocking some off because body surface area plays a part in the calculations as well as weight, and as weight goes up, surface area increases disproportionately less. But I had grown increasingly dissatisfied with this Heath Robinson approach to therapy. The textbooks on medicine give dose rates for a thousand and one drugs for man and animals, but never mention most of my patient species. Each kind of animal handles a drug, burns it up, destroys it, excretes it, at its own rate and that depends on its species, physiology, anatomy, size, speed of living and so on and so forth. I knew snakes were very slow clearers of most antibiotics, that guinea-pigs were strangely susceptible to poisoning by the safest antibiotic, penicillin, and that dolphins needed three times as much gentamycin, a broad-spectrum antibiotic, as a human of the same weight in order to maintain germ-killing levels in the blood. But for most drugs, many of which were potentially toxic in overdose, we didn't really know how much to give or how often to whales in order to do the job safely. With Freya, I decided to combine treatment and experimentation in a whale for the first time. 'We'll put Freya on to a course of amoxycillin,' I told John, 'and ask the laboratories to assay the levels of the drug in the blood at one, three, six, twelve and twenty-four hours after dosing. We know the levels of amoxycillin that are needed to kill sensitive bacteria, so if you sample Freya at those times we'll be able to calculate (a) whether the dose was right or needed to be adjusted, and (b) how long bug-killing levels are maintained.'

John was more than happy to collaborate, even though it meant him sampling during the night – his animals are his life – and we arranged for the blood samples to be sent by fast courier to specialist laboratories in France. The amoxycillin experiment went ahead at once, and we quickly obtained the information that gave us logical dosage levels and frequency for that drug in an average adult female killer whale. Unfortunately the amoxycillin didn't have any effect on the smouldering infection deep within Freya's body. So I switched to another antibiotic, cephalexin. Again we did the samplings and found the correct dosage level, but again the drug proved ineffectual in terms of curing the whale. After that came bacampicillin, lincomycin and doxycycline, with lots more samples for the labs to assay, but still the signs of infection advanced unchecked. It was some small consolation that we were getting information on the correct use of these drugs which should prove invaluable in the future.

Freya's lack of response to the treatment worried me deeply, and when, one day, she began to show signs of being off colour – listlessness and picking at her food – I flew out to France wondering what on earth to do next. I needed to know more about *where* the infection was situated. How could we get that information?

I had been involved with the Marineland at Antibes, Europe's finest, since before it opened in 1970. It was here I would bring Nemo and Limo, but the original stock of dolphins and sea lions came from Flamingo Park in Yorkshire where I was at the time resident as veterinary officer and assistant director, and Michael Riddell, the present director of Marineland, had trained with me when Cuddles, the first killer whale in Britain, arrived at Flamingo Park in 1969, and when, on Boxing Day of the same year, I brought the huge Calypso over from Canada for a short acclimatization period at Cleethorpes before going on to France. Marineland now has a large and ever-expanding marine animal complex with a ten-metre deep main whale pool, a breeding unit and crèche for king penguins, and lots of dolphins, seals and sea lions – including babies. Behind the scenes it is involved with the French government's attempts to save the highly endangered Mediterranean monk seal, marine fish breeding, and various scientific programmes concerned with the health of cetaceans. It was at Marineland that I had first 'washed' the blood of a sick killer whale with ozone, first tried, unsuccessfully, to X-ray the chest of a whale, first washed balls of leaves out of the stomach of a dolphin that had an obsession with the tidy collection of such floating plant material, and first looked inside a penguin's crop with a fibre-optic endoscope in search of a plastic feeder which it had swallowed. Other unique experiences for me on the French Riviera had included falling into an empty pool and damaging a shoulder which still hurts many years later and filming the second series of 'One By One' – in particular a sequence where the whale pool was awash with 'blood' (actually food colouring) and I was bitten by Miss Brigitte Bardot's favourite seal!

I went into discussion about Freya's deteriorating condition with Michael and John as soon as I arrived at Marineland, and we all walked round the hospital pool in which the whale was being held. She had obviously lost some weight: there was a distinct dip behind her head where there had once been plump, smooth blubber. Her appetite had now dropped to only a few kilograms of fish per day, taken with little enthusiasm. It was all horribly reminiscent of other killer whales which had suffered deep-seated, abscess-type infections. Most of them had been situated in the chest, either in the lungs themselves, or in the veil of tissue that separates the left chest from the right. A previous male whale at Marineland had developed just such a rugby-football-sized abscess in a gland at the border of the left lung, close to the ribs. The blood results, the bad smell from the animal's blow-hole and my instinct had all pointed to the infection being in the lung, but despite the use of high-powered industrial X-ray machines, we hadn't been able to locate and drain the abscess. The irony was that when I eventually post-mortemed the animal, I found the pus-filled cavity in a place where it would have been relatively easy to slip a large twelve-inch-long needle between the ribs in order to run off the foul liquid. Drainage, not just antibiotics, is essential in such cases, but you can't drain what you can't visualize!

'Freya could be just such another case,' I said to my friends.

'I *know* she's got a well-established infection of the soft tissues, and I'll bet my bottom dollar it's in the chest somewhere.'

'Do you want to try X-rays again?' asked Michael.

'X-rays aren't so good for soft lesions, but *if* we could get a reasonably good picture of the lungs, it should show up an abscess. Our last attempt however, was a failure, as you well know.'

Whales are so big and broad, padded with a dense layer of blubber, that portable X-ray machines just don't have the power to penetrate them. Even the biggest machines, such as those installed at the veterinary teaching hospitals, have major difficulties with horse chests and abdomens.

Michael is an unfailingly willing tryer, even if there's only the most outside of chances, and he's a brilliant fixer. 'There's a bloke in Nice with a new portable industrial X-ray that can find flaws in aircraft engines,' he said. 'I'm sure I could persuade him to bring the thing here, if you are interested.'

'Let's try it,' I replied. 'Nothing ventured . . .'

The hospital pools at Marineland make medical work with the whales and dolphins much easier than in some other establishments. These pools can be drained and refilled quickly, several times a day if necessary, and I can get at my patients 'in the dry' as they lie on the bottom. The man with the industrial X-ray machine arrived that evening, and he began setting up the device while explaining how it could find a hair-line fracture in a block of steel the size of a man's head. 'I weel put eem 'ere on ze right side of ze whale wiz ze X-ray source over ze lung wherever you want 'eem,' he said. 'Zen you put ze plates wiz ze X-ray film on ze left side, and I press ze button. *Zut!* You weel 'ave ze picture, I promise!' We covered the whole of Freya's left chest with X-ray film plates, held in place with adhesive tape.

'*Eh bien*! Stand clear – I now press ze button!' shouted the X-ray man. '*Voilà!*' A motor cyclist took the plates to the local hospital for development. Twenty minutes later he returned with the wet films – they were blank. 'Eet ees eempossible!' exclaimed the X-ray man. '*Encore!* We do eem again!' We did 'eem' again, and again the developed films showed not a single shadow. X-rays had again proved useless for our whales. One week later a strange circular zone of inflamed skin developed on the right-hand side of Freya's chest – just where the machine had been focused. It dropped out eventually to form an ulcer, which three years later has still not fully healed. Experts deny it, but I'm absolutely sure it's a radiation burn.

Freya stopped eating altogether and lost more weight. The blood analyses began to show early kidney failure. 'Fill the hospital tank with fresh water for a few days,' I said, 'and tease, coax, cajole fish into her, any way you can – you know what it means if we have to begin force-feeding her!'

Michael and John knew the enormous difficulties well enough: trying to get a wooden gag into a whale's mouth in order to keep it open, avoiding the indignantly thrashing tail and snapping jaws, pushing fish down the throat with your shoulder up against the teeth and your arm crushed between gag and roof of the animal's mouth. Having a bucket full of mashed-up fish regurgitated into your face, being soaked to the skin with the cold water spray used to keep the beached whale moist, tired out when doing the feeding for the umpteenth time in the middle of the night. We'd all seen people badly injured when swept off their feet by a swing of a whale's tail or struck by a spat-out gag weighing twenty kilograms or more.

John and Bruce, the Number Two whale handler at Marineland, understood only too well the implications when I recommended avoiding force-feeding at all costs, and they set about persuading the whale by swimming with her, talking, stroking, tickling her lips with a fresh-thawed herring, mackerel or capelin, to accept the bare minimum of food.

'What now?' asked Michael, ever optimistic, even after the débâcle with the X-ray. 'How else do you think we can look inside her chest. Surgery?'

'No. The technology doesn't exist yet to keep her going with an open-chest operation. It's tricky enough even with dolphins.'

'And there's obviously no chance of putting her through a CAT or NMR scanner.'

If there had been a chance of squeezing so gigantic a beast through the aperture in one of those ultra-modern, enormously expensive diagnostic machines, Michael would surely have found someone willing to let us do it, and if we'd had to fly the whale by helicopter to Paris with a fighter escort, and then lower it into the hospital by demolishing the roof of the building, he would have wangled it somehow, no matter what it cost!

'There is ultra-sound,' I said, 'the sort of machine used on pregnant women, and increasingly on dolphins and other animals, to produce images by sonar. Trouble is they too aren't powerful enough to penetrate monsters like Freya.'

Michael's face lit up. 'So you want a really powerful ultra-sound machine? Maybe I can get Thomson to help us.'

'Thomson?'

'Yes. Thomson SNCF, the French electronics company. Their military sonar research place is a few miles away from here, at Sophia Antipolis, the Silicon Valley of southern France. I'll get us an appointment to see a boffin!'

And, of course, he did.

A few hours later we drove up to the security post outside the Thomson complex and, after having our passports screened ('Being Englishmen makes you more risky as visitors than if you were Russian,' said the security man when he'd made several phone calls), we were led through long corridors to the door of a laboratory that bore a red sign with the French equivalent of 'Warning! Restricted Entry.'

'Wait here for a moment,' said our guide, 'we must wipe the blackboard clean of calculations before you enter.' When all the abstruse formulae had been obliterated, we were allowed to enter and were introduced to two scientists working in a clutter of flickering oscilloscope tubes and arcane electronic gadgets.

'*Messieurs*,' said Michael, 'as you know, we are from Marineland. And we have a problem with which you may be able to assist us. We need to look inside a whale's chest.' He explained Freya's condition, and what we would like to do.

The two men listened intently and then, when he had finished, one said, 'We do have naval sonar units of the required power, but to do what you require would mean, say, putting the whale into the water in Antibes harbour, and beaming the ultra-sound at her from a kilometre away out to sea. Treating her like a submarine. Hardly practical.'

'How much detail could we expect if we risked placing her in a sling in the harbour?' I asked.

The scientist smiled gently and made a typically Gallic gesture with his hands. 'We cannot reveal the resolution obtainable by our equipment in military applications. And as for the flesh of a whale, who knows?'

'What do you suggest, then?' I asked.

'Give us a week. We will try modifying one of our portable machines, and build a special probe, waterproof of course. Then we'll come to Marineland and try it out with the probe against the whale's skin.'

Michael and I were pleased with our 'penetration' of the Thomson sonar lab, and I felt sure I could keep Freya going for at least another week. We went back to Marineland, and I made arrangements for the whale to receive regular injections of vitamins and anabolic hormones prior to the ultra-sound scanning.

Seven days later I returned to Antibes on the usual BA flight, full of loaded gentlefolk, gold-medallioned poseurs and Panama-hatted City types accompanied by pale wives, nannies and fractious kids. I found Freya looking worse than ever. The two Thomson boffins arrived punctually at the agreed hour with a vanload of equipment and, while they set it up on a platform beside the hospital pool, John lowered the water level until the whale was barely afloat. The special probe, the size and shape of a paperback book, and connected to the ultra-sound machine by a long cable, would be held against the animal's chest by one of our whale-handlers. The boffins, two consultant radiologists from nearby hospitals and I would stand above, in front of the machine's monitor screen, recording everything of interest both on video and Polaroid film.

The scanning began . Although the ultra-sound emissions were inaudible to human ears, it was noticeable at once that in certain positions the probe seemed to annoy the whale. Quite probably she could hear the irritating whine of the machine in a way that we could not. Very slowly, in accordance with instructions shouted down to them, John and his assistants moved the probe up and down, forwards and back, over the whale's rib-cage. My eyes were glued to the monitor.

Suddenly the patches of black and white, the bands, blobs and speckled areas, made sense. I could see, could recognize the design. For the first time ever human beings were looking at the organs contained within a living whale's body. There was the skin, the blubber, the muscles. The ribs stood out in cross-section. Beneath them was the lining of the thoracic cavity, a shimmering silver line, then a dark space, and finally the lung. I could see blood vessels and, farther back, the typical, sharply angled diaphragm of the whale, the liver and a portion of the stomach. While we watched, a pretty shower of silver confetti, fish in the stomach, was tossed up by the natural contractions of that organ. '*Fantastique!*' I shouted, slapping one of the Thomson men on the back.

Even the powerful Thomson machine could not send its beam through to the centre of Freya's chest, but as we watched, and grew more familiar with the sonar images, it became apparent that there *was* something abnormal inside the animal. Having viewed the video we made at the time on many occasions since then, I still consider the best description of what we saw, the lesion, is a 'dragon's head'. Between the ribs and the outside of the lung on the right-hand side of the whale there reared a miniature fire-breathing *Tyrannosaurus rex*, about the size of a grapefruit according to the scale on the monitor screen.

I discussed the 'dragon's head' with the radiologist. The

'fiery breath', 'gaping jaws', and other features of the image suggested adhesions, strands and nodules of fibrous tissue, and that, in turn, gave us a diagnosis. Freya had a form of chronic pleurisy.

This was a most heartening outcome for me. Chest abscesses could have proved hopelessly inaccessible for drainage, but with a more diffuse infection on the lung's outer surface, I could concentrate on re-doubling the attack by drug treatment, and begin to use the cortisone family of chemicals against the adhesions. Thomson's boffins with their submarine warfare secrets had achieved a spectacular result in the fight to save the life of a killer whale. To celebrate, Michael took the team up to Mougins for a memorable dinner at Roger Vergé's.

We continued the assaying of antibiotic levels in Freya's blood when I started giving her erythromycin (the drug most commonly used in treating cases of legionnaires' disease), and powerful shots of cortisone. Slowly her appetite began to pick up, and she started to swim around the hospital pool instead of hanging forlornly in one corner. Two weeks after the diagnosis of pleurisy the Thomson scientists came back, and we repeated the ultra-sound examination; the 'dragon's head' was still recognizable, but it was clearly smaller in size and had begun to fragment. As time went by Freya's improvement was maintained and eventually she went back to the whale pool and her friends, her weight restored, eating with gusto and keen to join in the shows.

We continue to check the killer whale regularly, and I still don't consider her to be absolutely one hundred per cent normal, the healed scars in her chest cavity probably niggling her from time to time. But with any luck it will be many years before I see her lungs with my naked eye, thanks to the glimpses of them that I've had by means of the marvellous machine that turns inaudible soundwaves into pictures.

12 Baboons and Busybodies

> If you don't pay no mind to diseases, they will go away.
> James Thurber, *The Thurber Carnival*

One of the more curious aspects of the lunatic fringe of Animal Liberationists is that they often seem to relish killing animals. It may, of course, have been simple invincible ignorance when, for example, a bunch of these fanatics 'liberated' a large number of mink from a mink farm (a kind of establishment which I find distasteful, to say the least) and in so doing opened a Pandora's box: for the mink, ferocious little creatures, at once set about slaughtering any animal, from chicken to kitten, that they came upon in the surrounding countryside, and not because they were hungry. From time to time these people threaten, even attempt, to kill animals in zoos, to 'liberate' them, I suppose, from this mortal coil. Once slug pellets were thrown into a dolphin pool on the assumption that the animals would swallow them with toxic effects; and I have known several cases where Animal Liberationists have set fire to zoo buildings, with animals inside, to 'draw attention to the scandal of creatures in captivity'.

So when the Chairman of Windsor Safari Park received a call one evening to say that Animal Liberationists had poisoned the Park's baboons, all in the good cause, I was not unduly surprised. Half a dozen baboons, mainly females and youngsters, had indeed been found dead and dying that morning, but by the time the phone call was made, my assistant John Lewis and I were already convinced that the cause was something far more deadly than publicity-seeking petty criminals; the Animal Liberationists had simply jumped on the bandwagon after hearing of the incident, and had tried to take the perverted credit for something they did not do.

All the baboons, around ninety in number, had been fit and lively on the Friday evening. When the keepers arrived at the new baboon reserve at a quarter past eight on the Saturday morning, they found six corpses in the night-house. Three other baboons looked very ill. An hour later John and I arrived at the Safari Park, and went straight to see the sick animals.

I find baboons, such as the Hamadryas species at Windsor, in many ways the most interesting of primates. They look more 'human' than other monkeys, can pull all sorts of faces, are intelligent and sociable, and live in groups with a complex hierarchy. This is the baboon whose name comes from the Greek for 'wood nymph', that was worshipped by the ancient Egyptians as Anubis, that was thought, in the seventeenth century, to be half man and half animal, and whose long, straight muzzle may have given rise to the belief that dog-headed men existed. Adult male Hamadryas are brave and formidable individuals armed with dagger-like fang teeth. They will defend their family and friends against the most dangerous of predators, and even lions and leopards generally steer well clear of them. The vet working in the open on an injured or otherwise incapacitated baboon has to keep an eye peeled for other baboons who will come rushing to the rescue, hairy and furious like ancient Norse berserkers.

John and I stood in the porch of the baboons' night-house and watched the animals. Most were expectantly waiting for their door to be opened so that they could swarm out on to the reserve where they would spend the day busily playing, sorting out their domestic disputes, foraging for seeds and beetles in the grass and, as ever, contemplating ways of escaping into the surrounding forests that belong to Her Majesty The Queen. When the Billy Smart family had owned the park, the baboons had tried clinging on beneath the chassis of motor coaches and riding out as stowaways. They'd mastered the art of giving one another a leg-up or forming small baboon pyramids to overcome electrified wire, and they devised a way of diverting the attention of a noisy Alsatian running on a long leash at the gate, by sending one of their number to tease it, while the main band of absconders slipped through unnoticed by the preoccupied dog.

Windsor's baboons in those days had been expert auto-mechanics, able to strip the rubber seals off windscreens with a few quick picks of their hard and muscular fingers, thus enabling the glass to fall out, and they collected a garageful of accessories each season: aerials, hub-caps and windscreen wipers. The vultures who shared the old baboon reserve with them appreciated the monkeys' acquisitive tendencies, particularly towards the aerials and wipers, for they in turn picked them up and used them as nest-building materials when the baboons had finished playing with them.

It must be fun to be a baboon. On this particuar morning, the animals seemed as optimistic and impatient as usual – except for a handful that had the appearance of being hung-over. We caught them and examined them closely. No symptoms other than tired weakness – they were all the same – and when the others were released into the reserve, they would have preferred to stay behind, like humans who needed to catch up on sleep after a night on the town, but the bossy males wouldn't let them. They took them by hand, or threw an arm round their shoulders, and bustled them out.

Once in the reserve, where the sun was already strong, it being the middle of the hot summer of 1989, the ailing baboons became rapidly weaker before our eyes, and individuals full of *joie de vivre* only minutes before began to slow down dramatically as if all energy was draining from them, melted in the heat.

'Let's go and post-mortem the ones that died during the night,' I said to John, 'then we'll come back and perhaps be in a better position to do something for these.' Already, with six dead and as many ill, it was as bad an epidemic of *something* as I could remember in the twenty years since I'd taken my Royal College Fellowship in the Diseases of Primates.

The cadavers of the dead baboons were waiting for us in the post-mortem room. Gloved up, and with liberal quantities of iodine disinfectant to hand, we began the dissections, working at opposite ends of the table from each other. John had done his PhD on human tumours at the Charing Cross Hospital and, after working with us in Arabia for a year, had been veterinary pathologist at London Zoo. I had done human pathology after graduating in 1956. Both of us remain keen on this modern, scientific version of the old Roman sooth-sayer's art of haruspication – divination by the inspection of animals' entrails. All of the six baboons had an identical post-mortem appearance. Full stomachs, no visible signs of disease. But, as with Sherlock Holmes' curious incident of the dog in the night, such absence of evidence was evidence in itself. We could rule out heat-stroke and acute septicaemias, blood poisonings caused by germs that can cause rapid death. We took samples of stomach contents, blood, muscle and major organs for laboratory tests, and then scrubbed up and drove back to the baboon reserve.

'Could be malicious poisoning, perhaps,' said John, 'though it's difficult to see what and how.' I told him about the many such poisonings I'd seen in zoos, including the spate of incidents many years ago at Chester Zoo where a member of the staff had been strongly suspected of being the culprit. 'The majority of my poisoning cases have been with barbiturates of one kind or another – often sleeping pills,' I added. 'At least death from those drugs is painless. Not so for the dolphin at Rio León in Spain that was killed by a hazelnut-sized crystal of copper sulphate secreted inside a herring!'

Two more baboons had died and eight were lying sprawled on the ground when we reached the reserve. Again the symptoms were the same, and as sparse, in all the affected animals. Nothing dramatic, no diarrhoea, no vomiting, no blood, no pain, no fever – just weakness, progressing rapidly to death. We paid particular attention to their faces. No pin-point pupils in the eyes, nor the extreme dilatation that might signify barbiturate overdose. Just a drool of saliva along the lips. We took blood to look for the presence of poison, although for me it just didn't *feel* like a case of poisoning. 'They are having difficulty swallowing,' said John, pointing to a string of saliva.

'I've never seen it in primates,' I replied, 'but the more I look at these poor little devils, the more I think of botulism.'

John nodded vigorously. 'Just what I was thinking. Hot weather. Nothing to see in the post-mortems. No signs of gastro-enteritis that might be caused by salmonella or something like that.'

'In which case, we'd better start hunting for a source in the reserve straight away!'

Botulism is one of the most deadly forms of food poisoning. Though caused by a bacterium that multiplies in putrefying organic matter, particularly of animal origin, it isn't an infection, but an intoxication. The germ itself is ubiquitous and, given high temperature and humidity together with a suitable decaying food stuff, it will begin producing a chemical poison that is one of the most powerful known to science. It is the poison, persisting even if the bacteria themselves are destroyed, that causes the rapidly lethal effects through paralysing the motor nerves of the body. Human outbreaks are uncommon, but have been associated with such things as contaminated meat- or fish-paste and, recently, in the United Kingdom, hazelnut yoghurt. In periods of drought when water levels in ponds and rivers fall, and the quantity of dissolved oxygen is unusually low, birds may feed on maggots that have themselves picked up the toxin from dead fish and other creatures; and because the poison is soluble in water it can likewise contaminate water sources. Recent hot summers in Britain have seen wildfowl and swans dying from the disease in the Norfolk Broads and the royal parks of London. My experience of botulism was limited to cases in birds, and to an outbreak handled by Andrew which had involved circus lions fed on contaminated chickens.

No botulism expert, I nevertheless felt reasonably convinced that it was the likeliest explanation for the baboon deaths. To prove it, I sent the samples by courier to several laboratories among those that are prepared to work with primate material. (Many, including some government ones, will no longer touch monkey or ape material for fear that it might contain one of

the 'new' and often lethal viruses, such as that of Lassa fever
or B virus, that have come out of the African forests in recent
years.) Just in case I was wrong, I also sent it to one that
would look for poisons.

With Paul, the curator, we walked around the baboon
reserve looking for left-overs of anything that the animals
might have been eating on the previous day. Their standard
diet was vegetables, fruit, bread, dried rice and cereals. Sometimes surplus cooked meats from the cafeteria, unsold at the
end of the day, were sent down to the baboons; in winter I
am particularly keen that they should regularly be fed beef or
chicken incorporated in a specially cooked and delicious-
smelling stew that also contains onions and carrots. Searching
in the reserve we found some roasted sausages, boiled ham
and the scattered remains of the rice and cereal mix. Of course,
as I said to my colleagues, it was more than possible that
whatever might have caused the trouble had been totally
consumed by the baboons and was now just part of the mush
of stomach contents in our sample bottles. Only a tiny quantity
of contaminated food is enough to cause trouble; no more than
two little maggots carrying botulism toxins are sufficient to
snuff the life out of a wild duck. The sausages, ham and grain
we recovered were bagged and sent to the lab.

Treatment of the sick and the so far apparently unaffected
baboons was now our main concern, but there isn't much you
can do for those already showing symptoms. The iron lungs
that are employed with paralysed human botulism patients
can't help our animals. Botulism anti-toxin isn't available
commercially in this country, so when he'd been treating his
lions, Andrew had imported, under licence with the Ministry
of Agriculture, a quantity of anti-toxin from the United States.
We still possessed some, though it was theoretically out of
date.

A welter of regulations, the delight of the apparatchiks of
governmental bureaucracy, restrict what doctors or vets can
do with medicines that have to be obtained from abroad when
you want to use them. Though they can be imported under

licence, they must only be used, according to the grey men from the ministries, on the species specified in the licence. Caring little and knowing less about baboons or any other non-farmable, non-domesticated animal, such functionaries do at least know that a baboon is not a lion. When I spoke to the Ministry of Agriculture about my suspected cases of botulism and mentioned in passing that I intended to use our small stock of American anti-toxin on them, a quaint conversation ensued.

'You can't do that without a licence,' said the grey man.

'The baboons are dying, and I'm going to try to protect as many of the so far unaffected ones as possible, after treating the sick individuals with it.'

'You'll need a modification to the licence.'

'Today is Saturday. They're dying as I speak.'

'We should be able to issue the modification on Monday.'

'Big deal!'

'The licence was issued for anti-toxin to be used on *lions* by your partner.'

'This is an *emergency*! These are *real* animals, not statistics on off-white ministry paper. I'm responsible for them. I want to use the anti-toxin. *Now*.'

'No need to sound so cantankerous, Dr Taylor. I'm sure everything can be sorted out on Monday. Use on other species of such material without licence is a prosecutable offence.'

'Go ahead and prosecute. I'm treating them with it within five minutes!'

We used what anti-toxin we had and, though it slowed the course of the disease in the sick baboons, they still died. I worried about whether my diagnosis was correct. 'Treatment of botulism in animals is often said to be virtually hopeless,' said John, when I aired my doubts. 'And maybe the anti-toxin had lost its potency. I'm sure we're on the right track.'

By the Monday twenty baboons were dead, and still others were showing symptoms. On Tuesday the total was thirty-five, but there were no new cases. Wednesday brought the total mortality figure up to forty-two. Thereafter no more deaths or cases of illness occurred. At breakfast time on Wednesday morning the phone rang. It was one of the bacteriology laboratories to which I had sent samples. 'The baboon blood was full of botulism toxin,' said the microbiologist who had done the tests. 'It killed white mice within minutes. And we found it in the stomach contents, too. Mouse protection tests prove it to be botulism Type C. There's no news yet about the possible source. We're still trying to grow the bug from all the samples you sent.' I was relieved that at last we knew for sure the nature of the epidemic. During its five-day course the bodies of almost half of the Windsor baboon colony, the biggest in Britain, had been sent to the incinerators, by far the worst holocaust in my career with exotic animals.

By a week later the laboratories had found the botulism germ in some of the boiled ham samples we'd sent in. Puzzled, for the ham in the cafeteria was of the highest quality, hygienically handled, and had been shown to be free of bacterial contamination, I made further detailed inquiries as to what happened to the surplus meat when it left the kitchens for the baboon reserve. The last piece of the jigsaw fell into place when I discovered that, on the day before the outbreak began, someone had made a fundamental mistake. They had given the baboons ham that had lain, contrary to the normal strict procedures, for three or four days in a closed, black, plastic bag exposed to the unusually hot weather. Botulism bacteria in particles of soil within the bag had multiplied enthusiastically in the warm humid conditions, while feeding on the ham. Human error, as so often the case in such isolated incidents, had exacted a terrible price amongst some of humans' not too distant relatives.

Baboons had been at the centre of a quite different sort of problem at Belle Vue Zoo twenty-five years before. It happened during the time when, for a few months, Matt Kelly was acting superintendent. He telephoned me one breakfast time, clearly in a state of considerable exasperation. 'Moi office has been occupied,' he announced hoarsely, 'by a pride of . . . of women! Sittin' in me room. Won't budge, bejasus. And they've talked me to a standstill!' Now that *was* a serious matter; the ever-loquacious Irishman, whose words could charm anything on two or four legs, *out-talked*! My curiosity burned bright as I waited for him to clear his throat and continue.

'These . . . these . . . ladies have a complaint—' Matt sounded as if he were about to spit into the telephone. 'A complaint, bhoy, a whole barrowload of complaints.'

'About what, Matt?' I interjected.

'You moit well ask. It's the baboons, and one of the black apes, and the mandrills in particular and . . . and . . . You've got to come down.'

'But what are they complaining about?' For its day, Belle Vue's monkey collection and colony of baboons were among the healthiest, best-housed and most fecund in the country. I couldn't imagine what . . .

'Oi can't say on the phone. Oi . . . oi . . . it's . . .'

Curiouser and curiouser. Matt was never one to mince words.

'Well, is it some incident of what they imagine is poor management, or an injury, or an illness they've spotted?'

'No . . . Please, David me bhoy, come down.'

'I will, but can't you give me a clue?'

'The . . . the ladies . . . are sitting here as oi speak. Errr . . . oi can't say no more.'

'But are any of the animals in trouble? Do I need anything special – drugs or instruments?'

'No. Just come down, me bhoy. It's . . . it's sort of a moral . . . moral . . .'

'Dilemma?'

'Doilemma – yes, one of those. The ladies, the darlin' ladies, have been infected with a doilemma.'

Highly intrigued, I took my 'Woodhouse', the favourite toasted sandwich loaded with bacon, tomato, mustard and Worcester sauce, that Shelagh and I had named after the Jacobean farmhouse in which we lived, and went out to the car. What on earth was the 'moral dilemma' that had apparently so flabbergasted the experienced head keeper cum superintendent? Munching my breakfast I drove the familiar route, more or less the same one that I'd taken when going to school in Manchester from the age of ten. Down through Heywood, the place we used to call 'monkey town' because it was said that all the stools in the pubs in that town had holes in the centre through which the inhabitants could let down their tails, through Middleton, passing the pet shop where once my daughter, Stephanie, and I had been cornered by a spitting cobra, up Bogart Hall Clough to Blackley, and then left between rows of blackened terraced houses, to arrive at last at the gates of the great park with its speedway, ballrooms, exhibition halls, pubs, funfair, old brewery, railway sidings, firework island and, most magical of all to generations of folk born and bred in Greater Manchester, its zoo, still with a Victorian elephant house and sea-lion pool.

Forty minutes after he'd spoken to me on the telephone, Matt opened the door of his office at my first knock.

'Come in – glad ye're here.' He was now the relaxed, courteous, smiling Matt I knew so well. The superintendent's office was not large, its volume being further reduced by bookcases bursting with old zoological tomes and the bound records of Belle Vue's long history. Shelves and walls were cluttered with bleached skulls, bundles of exotic bird feathers, dusty, stuffed animals and mounted antelope horns. At the far end in the light of a corner window was the heavy mahogany desk. This morning, sitting on chairs in front of him, were three middle-aged ladies. The trio were of similar medium height and matronly build. All were wearing dark coats and dark hats. Matt steered me towards a chair next to his facing the women across the desk and introduced me. 'And these ladies are . . .'

'Mrs Schofield.'

'Miss Ogden.'

'Miss Butterworth.'

They identified themselves crisply.

'Now the situation, David,' said Matt, 'is that these good ladies want action boi me . . . us . . . on a matter that has me banjaxed. They see a problem with the baboons that just isn't a problem.'

Miss Butterworth, her round and curiously flattened face with small black eyes resembling that of a gingerbread man before baking, wagged a gloved finger vigorously.

'Mr Kelly, it really is outrageous for you to pretend there is no cause for concern, serious concern.' Her high piping voice was that of a child. Her companions nodded, and crossing their arms under their bosoms, hitched them upwards in unison, a movement that seemed to signify their resolute solidarity with the speaker. 'It's a matter of morals, of civilized behaviour,' she continued, 'of the effect these creatures will undoubtedly have on children, and God-fearing, well-brought-up adults.'

'The rate-payers of Manchester,' chipped in Mrs Schofield, thick-rimmed spectacles perched far down her aquiline nose.

'Wholesome Christian values under siege as ever by the legions of permissiveness,' said Miss Ogden, in a broad Lancashire accent, barely opening her thin-lipped, perfectly straight slot of a mouth.

'The Old Adam!' trilled Miss Butterworth cryptically.

'I'm sorry, but you'll have to explain,' I said, looking at Matt. 'Is this a veterinary matter?' He made a sort of grating noise and then clicked his teeth.

'Oi think oi'll leave it to the ladies to state the nature of their grievance.'

Miss Butterworth fumbled in her handbag and brought out a small Bible. Clasping it in both hands she directed her eyes, currants in a circle of pale dough, at me.

'It's a subject of considerable embarrassment, not to say lewdness,' she began. 'There are monkeys in Belle Vue, baboons, and most notably the mandrills, that should not be on show to the public.'

'Why not?' I asked.

Miss Ogden and Mrs Schofield were both looking down fixedly at their crossed arms.

'Because . . . because . . . they are, quite simply, *obscene.*'

Heads still down, her companion nodded in agreement.

'In what way can animals be obscene?'

Matt lay back in his chair, eyes closed and with a faint smile on his lips. Obviously he'd gone through all this earlier on.

'It is because they are blatantly displayed, rudely displayed – for visitors, mothers, children, impressionable youths, to see.'

'But what exactly do you mean?'

There was a faint squawk from Matt, which I imagined was an imperfectly suppressed guffaw.

'It is a zoo's responsibility to see that animals do not flaunt, do not disgust the public with . . . with their *pudenda.*'

'You mean their sex organs. And they don't, except for man, wear clothes to cover them.'

'We realize that, Dr Taylor. And I should emphasize that my friends here and I are all animal-lovers, as well as being workers for the Greater Manchester Christian Crusade. We have cats. Miss Ogden has a budgerigar. Our complaint, our insistence, is that certain monkeys here flaunt their . . . things . . . in a most promiscuous way, and that the zoo does nothing, has done nothing over the months we have been monitoring the lamentable state of affairs, and despite several letters from the Crusade and Mrs Lumb, our pastor, to attend to these creatures.'

'*Attend* to them?'

'Yes. It cannot be normal for that monkey, the mandrill I believe it is called, to have such an excessively, artificially, red and blue face and red . . . posterior.'

'Quite!' murmured Miss Ogden.

'And the way the male mandrills and baboons . . . exhibit themselves . . . in a condition of . . . excitement and . . . abuse themselves so frequently, must indicate they are all psychopathically abnormal. There's a black monkey that is positively perverted! And all of their depraved antics can be *seen by unsuspecting visitors.*'

'Shocking,' averred Mrs Schofield.

'So we demand that something be done,' continued Miss Butterworth. 'As the people responsible for the animals here, Mr Kelly and you should take these unsavoury beasts off display until you have treated the problem successfully. I must say, Dr Taylor, that as veterinary surgeon here you seem to have been wilfully lax in neglecting this problem for so long.'

She was of course, right – up to a point. Our baboons enjoyed an uninhibited sex life, just like baboons always have, and the male mandrills' startling colours, perfectly normal in mature adults, did add a certain dramatic quality to these handsome animals' frequent priapic revels. There was indeed a Celebes black ape (actually a kind of monkey) who hated men but adored women, and would try to entice a female visitor to stretch out her hand towards him by winsome looks and friendly gestures, and who, when she responded, would shoot an arm out through the mesh and take hold of her sleeve while masturbating with his other hand. He *was* rather odd, having been raised originally as a pet and then given to the zoo when he became a difficult adult. But he'd never harmed anyone.

Most people ignored or smiled at the animals' Rabelaisian behaviour; although there were some, elderly ladies in the main, who seemed utterly fascinated by what went on. Several came regularly to eat sandwiches on one of the benches outside an exhibit where such things could be guaranteed to occur. We had observed that in other parts of the zoo, the couplings of the tapirs and hippopotamuses were also popular among such silver-haired voyeuses.

One thing was certain – we could, and would, do nothing about these displays of natural behaviour.

'I'm afraid that I cannot go along with your attitude towards these things, ladies,' I said. 'If you think monkeys are promiscuous, you ought to watch our tortoises in summer or dolphins in one of the new marinelands! Where would it all end if we began trying to interfere in such areas of animal biology?'

'For one thing, we'd have no more babies!' interrupted Matt.

'And anyway, there's nothing I could do even if I wanted to suppress their normal inclinations.' Actually that wasn't quite true – in individual cases of sexual aggressiveness in males of various species, I was beginning to use the sort of drugs administered to sex criminals in order to diminish their libido. Nowadays I regularly prescribe such reversible anti-sex-hormone compounds for dangerously macho dolphins, antelopes or even ostriches, if they go around beating up their weaker brethren.

'Surely you could "doctor" them?' suggested Miss Ogden.

'We *breed* our animals, missus!' replied Matt, rather irascibly.

'Well what about covering them up, or taking them off show during their lascivious moods?'

'Cover them?'

'Yes. Cover them. It's not impossible. The Crusade is gratified to hear that in America a campaign has been launched by like-minded Christians to cover up domestic animals of the more flagrant sort.' Matt's face, no longer smiling, was now an interesting shade of puce. He continually clicked his teeth and fiddled with a peacock feather taken from a vase on his desk.

'Coverin' animals? what sort of malarkey is that?' he muttered.

I'd read about it; in 1963 the Society for Indecency to (sic) Naked Animals was founded in the United States to promote the wearing of knickers by bitches and boxer shorts by dogs.

'Miss Butterworth!' I said. 'This really is all a waste of time. The idea of our monkeys wearing some sort of pantaloons or being castrated or doped or put off show is quite ridiculous. We, and the vast majority of visitors, like our animals the way they are. If you can't stand to see an animal naked in all its innocence and glory, then why not stay away from the zoo?'

For a short space of time the three women stared at us, saying nothing. Then Miss Butterworth suddenly waved her Bible at me. 'The Good Book!' she squeaked. 'It's all in here about corruption and lewdness and beasts. If you aren't prepared to put things right here we, the Crusade, will mount a campaign, write to the *Evening News*, warn our brethren and the citizens of Manchester not to come to the zoo. Purity must and will prevail. Mark my words, you'll see the number of your visitors fall like the Midianites.'

'So be it,' I replied. 'Do whatever you feel necessary.'

'Oi'm a Catholic, anyway,' said Matt.

Miss Butterworth glared at him and said, 'That explains it.' Which, of course, it didn't. There followed a long and awkward silence with much bosom-hitching by the women, who showed no signs of leaving.

Then, suddenly, Matt stood up; he was smiling gently once again. He walked over to a chest of drawers in which some of the zoo's curios were kept, and began routing about. Presently he returned to his desk carrying several objects. 'You talkin' about animals' sexual ways, ladies, got me thinkin'. In moi little museum here of zoological oddities and the loike, oi've got some bits and pieces that moit interest you.' He picked up a small bleached bone. 'D'ye know where this comes from, ladies? This here is the bone from the penis of a wolf! Oi use it in me lectures. Think of it, a penis with a real bone insoide!'

Three pairs of eyes bulged as they regarded the head keeper.

'And this,' – he now brandished a large molar tooth – 'this is scoientifically very interesting. It's a tooth, one that David here took out from a Przewalski's horse a couple of years back. But it didn't come out of its mouth. Oh no! He found it, would you believe, growing in one of its *testicles*. A tooth tumour that had made one testicle as big as a melon. Imagine! And here oi have . . .'

I watched him reach for the long, antique whip made from the phallus of a sperm whale.

'That's quite enough, Mr Kelly,' cried Miss Butterworth in a surprisingly loud treble, 'quite enough. I can see that unholy vulgarity permeates the fabric of this place. Come along Marjorie, Ruth.' She rose. Her companions followed. Matt hurried to show them out.

When he had closed the door behind them we looked at one another, and began to laugh like unhinged hyenas.